Microbiology and Infection Prevention and Control for Nursing Students

SAGE was founded in 1965 by Sara Miller McCune to support the dissemination of usable knowledge by publishing innovative and high-quality research and teaching content. Today, we publish over 900 journals, including those of more than 400 learned societies, more than 800 new books per year, and a growing range of library products including archives, data, case studies, reports, and video. SAGE remains majority-owned by our founder, and after Sara's lifetime will become owned by a charitable trust that secures our continued independence.

Los Angeles | London | New Delhi | Singapore | Washington DC | Melbourne

Microbiology and Infection Prevention and Control for Nursing Students

Deborah Ward

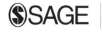

Los Angeles | London | New Delhi
Singapore | Washington DC

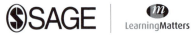

Learning Matters
An imprint of SAGE Publications Ltd
1 Oliver's Yard
55 City Road
London EC1Y 1SP

SAGE Publications Inc.
2455 Teller Road
Thousand Oaks, California 91320

SAGE Publications India Pvt Ltd
B 1/I 1 Mohan Cooperative Industrial Area
Mathura Road
New Delhi 110 044

SAGE Publications Asia-Pacific Pte Ltd
3 Church Street
#10-04 Samsung Hub
Singapore 049483

Editor: Alex Clabburn
Development editor: Eleanor Rivers
Production controller: Chris Marke
Project management: Swales & Willis Ltd,
Exeter, Devon
Marketing manager: Camille Richmond
Cover design: Wendy Scott
Typeset by: C&M Digitals (P) Ltd, Chennai, India
Printed and bound by CPI Group (UK) Ltd,
Croydon, CR0 4YY

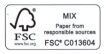

MIX
Paper from
responsible sources
FSC   FSC® C013604
www.fsc.org

First published 2016

Library of Congress Control Number: 2015955830

British Library Cataloguing in Publication data

A catalogue record for this book is available from the
British Library

ISBN 978-1-4739-2534-2
ISBN 978-1-4739-2535-9 (pbk)

At SAGE we take sustainability seriously. Most of our products are printed in the UK using FSC papers and boards.
When we print overseas we ensure sustainable papers are used as measured by the PREPS grading system.
We undertake an annual audit to monitor our sustainability.

Contents

Transforming Nursing Practice is a series tailor-made for pre-registration student nurses. Each book in the series is:

- Affordable
- Mapped to the NMC Standards and Essential Skills Clusters
- Full of active learning features
- Focused on applying theory to practice

Each book addresses a core topic and they have been carefully developed to be simple to use, quick to read and written in clear language.

> An invaluable series of books that explicitly relates to the NMC standards. Each book cover a different topic that students need to explore in order to develop into a qualified nurse... I would recommend this series to all Pre-Registration nursing students whatever their field or year of study
>
> **Linda Robson**
> **Senior Lecturer, Edge Hill University**
>
> The set of books is an excellent resource for students. The series is small, easily portable and valuable. I use the whole set on a regular basis.
>
> **Fiona Davies**
> **Senior Nurse Lecturer, University of Derby**
>
> I recommend the SAGE/Learning Matters series to all my students as they are relevant and concise. Please keep up the good work.
>
> **Thomas Beary**
> **Senior Lecturer in Mental Health Nursing, University of Hertfordshire**

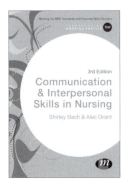

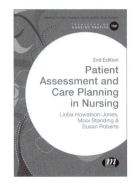

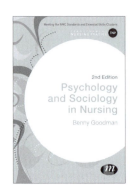

About the author

Dr Deborah Ward began her healthcare career in 1990 working in the NHS. Since then she has had various roles, becoming interested in infection prevention and control as a speciality while working on a regional tropical and infectious diseases unit between 1996 and 1998. After that, she began a career as an infection prevention and control nurse working in both hospital and primary care settings, both inside the NHS and in the private sector. Latterly, she went to work at the University of Manchester as a lecturer in infection prevention and control in 2007, teaching a variety of subjects including infection prevention and control and microbiology at both undergraduate and postgraduate level.

Acknowledgements

A big thank you to Dr Andrea Denton, Senior Lecturer in Adult Nursing, Acute and Critical Care, University of Huddersfield, for acting as peer reviewer for this book.

I would also like to acknowledge the reproduction of the NPSA/NHS poster in Chapter 8, page 124 under the following licence: www.nationalarchives.gov.uk/doc/open-government-licence/version/3/

I would also like to thank Eleanor Rivers from Learning Matters for her support throughout the process of writing this book.

Introduction

About this book/Who is this book for?

This book is specifically aimed at nursing students undertaking a pre-registration undergraduate programme within the UK. It provides information about both microbiology and infection prevention and control which students will be able to use to assist them in meeting the Infection Control Essential Skills Cluster, to underpin their clinical practice and to aid their understanding of both the theory and practice relating to infection and its prevention in healthcare. Other healthcare students, such as pre-registration midwifery students, might also find this text useful.

Book structure

This book comprises nine chapters, each containing activities, scenarios, case studies and example multiple choice questions to encourage you to find additional information, apply the knowledge gained to practice and to test the knowledge that you have gained throughout the book.

Chapter 1 acts as an introduction to the subject, highlighting the problem of healthcare-associated infection and identifying some of the agencies and organisations which are of value for advice and further information during both your time as a student and throughout your career.

Chapter 2 introduces the concepts of microbiology and the chain of infection, providing initial information about aspects such as the routes of transmission, sources of infection and signs and symptoms of infection.

Chapter 3 covers bacteria, introducing you to the bacterial classification system, some of the bacterial infections which you may come across in practice and to the concept of antibiotic use.

Chapter 4 introduces you to viruses, identifying some of the viral infections which you may come across and considering treatment options.

Chapter 5 discusses fungi, parasites and prions, looking at their nature, some of the infections that they cause and how they might be treated.

Chapter 6 looks at microbiological specimens which are our way of identifying the micro-organisms causing infection and their treatment options. This chapter considers some of the specimens obtained and what tests might be undertaken.

Chapter 7 looks at the roles involved in infection prevention and control, such as members of the infection prevention and control team and what they do in practice.

Chapter 8 introduces you to the concepts of standard and transmission based precautions, focusing on hand hygiene, the use of protective clothing, sharps management, body fluid spillage management and decontamination.

Chapter 9, the final chapter, looks at infection prevention and control aspects such as isolation, uniform and workwear and aseptic technique, with a focus on urinary catheterisation and intravenous access devices.

Requirements for the NMC *Standards for Pre-registration Nursing Education* and the Essential Skills Clusters

The Nursing and Midwifery Council (NMC) has established standards of competence to be met by applicants to different parts of the register, and these are the standards it considers necessary for safe and effective practice. In addition to the competencies, the NMC has set out specific skills that nursing students must be able to perform at various points of an education programme. These are known as Essential Skills Clusters (ESCs). This book is structured so that it will help you to understand and meet the competencies and ESCs required for entry to the NMC register. The relevant competencies and ESCs are presented at the start of each chapter so that you can clearly see which ones the chapter addresses. There are *generic standards* that all nursing students irrespective of their field must achieve, and *field-specific standards* relating to each field of nursing; i.e. mental health, children's health, learning disability and adult nursing. Each chapter refers to generic standards which are applicable to all fields of study within nursing.

This book includes the latest standards for 2010 onwards, taken from the *Standards for pre-registration nursing education* (NMC, 2010).

Learning features

Learning from reading text is not always easy. Therefore, to provide variety and to assist with the development of independent learning skills and the application of theory to practice, this book contains activities, case studies, scenarios, further reading, useful websites and other materials to enable you to participate in your own learning. You will need to develop your own study skills and 'learn how to learn' to get the best from the material. The book cannot provide all the answers, but instead provides a framework for your learning.

The activities in the book will in particular help you to make sense of, and learn about, the material being presented. Some activities ask you to reflect on aspects of practice, or your experience of it, or the people or situations you encounter. *Reflection* is an essential skill in nursing, and it helps you understand the world around you and often to identify how things might be improved. Other activities will help you develop key graduate skills such as your ability to *think critically* about a topic in order to challenge received wisdom, or your ability to *research a topic and find appropriate information and evidence,* and to be able to *make decisions* using that evidence in situations that are often difficult and time-pressured. Communication and working as part of a team are core to all nursing practice, and some activities will ask you to carry out *team work activities* or think about your *communication skills* to help develop these. Finally, as a registered nurse you will be expected to *lead and manage* your own team, case load or area of care, and so some activities focus on helping you build confidence in doing this.

All the activities require you to take a break from reading the text, think through the issues presented and carry out some independent study, possibly using the internet. Where appropriate, there are sample answers presented at the end of each chapter, and these will help you to under-stand more fully your own reflections and independent study. Remember, academic study will always require independent work; attending lectures will never be enough to be successful on your programme, and these activities will help to deepen your knowledge and understanding of the issues under scrutiny and give you practice at working on your own.

You might want to think about completing these activities as part of your personal development plan (PDP) or portfolio. After completing the activity write it up in your PDP or portfolio in a section devoted to that particular skill, then look back over time to see how far you are developing. You can also do more of the activities for a key skill that you have identified a weakness in, which will help build your skill and confidence in this area.

This book also contains a glossary on page 171 to assist you with unfamiliar terms. Glossary terms are in **bold** in the first instance that they appear.

We hope that you find this book stimulating and useful in your studies, both in the university setting and in practice with your patients. You might also find it useful in normal life, as people do get infections outside of the hospital setting which they might wish to ask you about during your studies.

Chapter 1
Background

Chapter aims

After reading this chapter you will be able to:

*   Highlight the extent of the problem of healthcare-associated infection both in the UK and internationally.
*   Discuss some of the consequences of healthcare-associated infection.
*   Identify some of the important organisations related to infection and its prevention and control in healthcare.

Introduction

In the UK, 5000 people a year die from healthcare-associated infections, with a further 15,000 deaths occurring with such infections as a contributory factor. Around 300,000 hospital infections occur each year. (Health Protection Agency, 2012a)

This chapter will introduce you to infection and healthcare-associated infection and its consequences. Firstly we will consider the effects on patients, then on healthcare staff such as nurses and finally on healthcare organisations. We then go on to discuss the various organisations available to provide information and support to nurses in relation to healthcare-associated infection, the websites for which are provided at the end of the chapter so that you are able to gain access to these before identifying relevant infection prevention and control related legislation. The end of this chapter looks at public health aspects of infection prevention and control. Throughout the chapter are case studies and activities which will enable you to link the information in the chapter with clinical practice as a nurse.

The last point **prevalence** survey in 2011 in England identified a healthcare-associated infection prevalence of 6.4% with the most common sites being the respiratory and urinary tracts and surgical sites (Health Protection Agency, 2012a). This means that 6.4% of patients admitted to hospital acquire an infection related to their admission. This is considered to be an estimate as many infections occur after discharge from hospital and these are not always identified in hospital statistics. Healthcare-associated (also called **nosocomial**) infections (HCAIs) are both a national and international issue. According to the European Centre for Disease Prevention and Control (ECDC, 2007) there are an estimated 50,000 deaths every year in Europe from HCAIs and 99,000 deaths every year in the US. HCAI, then, is clearly a global problem. It is estimated that between 15% and 30% of HCAIs are avoidable by the application of what we already know about infection prevention. In nursing we aim to minimise the risk of infection as far as we can to prevent avoidable infection in our patients. To do this we apply specific precautions, discussed later in Chapters 8 and 9. In the UK we are supported by various organisations and pieces of legislation in the form of information and advice, legal frameworks and guidance.

Consequences of healthcare-associated infections

HCAIs can have negative effects on patients, staff, healthcare services and the local community. It is important as nurses that we consider these consequences as they can be the direct or indirect result of our action or inaction in the healthcare environment. In order to consider consequences, they can be divided into those related to the patient, those related to staff and those which affect the healthcare organisation involved.

Effects on patients

Patients who acquire a HCAI (also referred to as nosocomial if specifically acquired in hospital) can suffer a range of associated consequences from relatively minor to so severe that they result in their death. They may have to stay in hospital for a longer period, be off work for longer or may even suffer permanent consequences such as a disability that means they can no longer work in their current job role or at all. If at home with an HCAI they may require additional services from the health and care sectors including their GP, district and practice nurses and their local pharmacist. There will often be delays in a return to a patient's normal level of function so that some patients require relatives to care for them at home. HCAIs also result in a poorer physical and mental health status.

Effects on staff

Effects on staff could be considered both as a consequence of caring for patients who may be more severely ill or for themselves if they acquire an infection through their work. When healthcare workers such as nurses acquire infections at work, they may need to be on sick leave which affects both them and their colleagues; the latter may need to work in an area where they are now short of staff or bank/agency staff may be required to cover the absent member of staff. For nurses who work full time for an agency, being on sick leave means that they do not earn their salary which clearly has financial implications for them. However, the risk of infection to staff is very small if infection prevention and control precautions are applied, as detailed in Chapters 8 and 9. When an infection occurs on a ward, for example, staff may feel guilty about whether the infection was avoidable. **Root cause analysis** is a process within healthcare that looks at the causes of an incident, such as an HCAI, and nurses may need to be involved in this process which can be worrying for them. There are also set targets within organisations for infection rates relating to some infections so the Infection Control Team (see Chapter 7) may be involved in investigating cases of HCAI which can also have consequences for nurses caring for patients.

Effects on the healthcare organisation

There is a potentially avoidable cost of £150 million per annum associated with HCAI in England, with each such infection costing an additional £4000–10,000 (National Audit Office, 2009). There are therefore financial costs associated with HCAI. Data on infections in England are regularly updated on the Public Health England website (see later for website). In addition to this, we need to consider costs to reputation.

In order to put these effects into context, it is worth considering a real situation.

Activity 1.1   *Reflection*

Consider what occurred at East Maidstone and Tunbridge Wells Trust in relation to an outbreak of *Clostridium difficile* by searching online. What do you think the consequences have been of the outbreak to this NHS Trust?

An outline answer is provided at the end of the chapter.

As you will have seen from your research around this event, the consequences were far-reaching, beyond even the affected organisation.

In terms of reputation, this might lead from newspaper or television reports related to HCAI in the local and national media as in the activity case above. The effects of negative attention such as this on an NHS organisation could be devastating in terms of commissioning and funding for future services. It is not within the remit of this book to discuss commissioning arrangements for services within the NHS, but funding for services that are not seen as meeting required standards or which patients no longer wish to access due to a poor reputation, could be severely restricted leading to scaling back or even closure of services.

Case study

Julian is a 32-year-old self-employed plumber. He is involved in a road traffic collision while out on his motorbike which has resulted in multiple fractures to his left tibia and fibula. He is admitted to an orthopaedic ward at his local hospital and undergoes surgery to pin the breaks in the operating theatre. Five days after his surgery his wound shows signs and symptoms of infection (discussed in Chapter 2) and his nurse obtains a wound swab to test for the presence of micro-organisms. The laboratory identifies the presence of bacteria and combined with his signs and symptoms this indicates a bacterial infection which needs to be treated with antibiotics.

Activity 1.2   *Critical thinking*

Consider the case study above. What are the possible effects of this infection on Julian, the hospital staff and the hospital as an organisation?

An outline answer is provided at the end of the chapter.

The above case study should have enabled you to consider the consequences and effects of healthcare-associated infection on an individual patient. In order to assist you in your role as a nurse when caring for such patients, there are various national and international organisations which provide support, in addition to local sources of information such as care plans, care pathways and local policies and procedures.

Important organisations in infection prevention and control

There are various organisations which can provide support for both healthcare workers such as nurses and the public. They can provide support and information, guidance and data on infection. These are a useful source of information for nursing students, both in academic work and in clinical practice.

Public Health England (PHE)

This is an executive agency supported by the Department of Health which aims to protect the nation's health and wellbeing and reduce health inequalities. It produces policies and guidelines related to HCAIs and other infections such as pandemic influenza guidance.

Health Protection Scotland

This is Scotland's organisation for public health and health protection. It has also published Scotland's national infection prevention and control manual which provides policies for Scottish healthcare organisations which they can use as a template for their own local policies.

Public Health Wales

This is the Welsh equivalent of Public Health England. It is also responsible for publication of National Infection Control Policies for Wales which act as a basis for policies in NHS organisations across Wales. It has links to several Public Health England guidelines, and also to Welsh guidelines such as their 2012 guidelines on the infection prevention and control management of patients with influenza.

Public Health Agency

This is the PHE equivalent in Northern Ireland. Though there is a template of infection prevention and control policies in Northern Ireland, these are not via the PHA and are instead accessible through a specific website (see the end of this chapter).

The NHS Commissioning Board Special Health Authority

The NPSA division transferred to this organisation in 2012 and it leads and contributes to improved, safe patient care by informing, supporting and influencing organisations and people working in the health sector.

They are an arm's length body of the Department of Health and through their divisions cover the UK health service. The Patient Safety Division aims to identify and reduce risks to patients receiving NHS care and leads on national initiatives to improve patient safety.

The Infection Prevention Society (IPS)

The IPS vision is that no person is harmed by a preventable infection. Their mission is to inform, promote and sustain expert infection prevention policy and practice in the pursuit of patient or service user and staff safety wherever care is delivered.

The IPS has three key aims. IPS will:

1. lead, shape and *inform* the infection prevention agenda locally, nationally and internationally;
2. influence and *promote* the evidence base for infection prevention practice that is adopted universally;
3. be the organisation of choice for all those involved in infection prevention to *sustain* improvements in practice.

The IPS provides publications and guidelines related to infection prevention such as commissioning and audit tools and quality improvement tools and has a professional publication – the *Journal of Infection Prevention* – which is published bi-monthly. This is a useful resource for nursing students in providing an evidence base for practice.

The Healthcare Infection Society (HIS)

This is a society for healthcare professionals working on prevention and control of healthcare-associated infections rather than nursing students, but their journal, the *Journal of Hospital Infection,* is a useful resource and they also produce guidelines such as those on the prevention of group A streptococcal infections, norovirus outbreak management and operating theatre standards.

The European Centre for Disease Prevention and Control (ECDC)

The European Centre for Disease Prevention and Control (ECDC) was established in 2005. It is an EU agency aimed at strengthening Europe's defences against infectious diseases. ECDC's mission is to identify, assess and communicate current and emerging threats to human health posed by infectious diseases.

In order to achieve this mission, the ECDC works in partnership with national health protection bodies across Europe to strengthen and develop continent-wide disease surveillance and early warning systems. By working with experts throughout Europe, ECDC pools Europe's health knowledge to develop authoritative scientific opinions about the risks posed by current and emerging infectious diseases.

Guidelines produced by ECDC include those relating to tuberculosis control, the introduction of the HPV (human papillomavirus) vaccine across Europe and HIV testing.

The Care Quality Commission (CQC)

The CQC is the regulator of all health and social care services in England, including those provided by both the NHS and the private sector. These include hospitals, care homes, dentists, clinics, GPs, home care agencies, mental health and learning disability services and other community and home services related to health and social care. The CQC inspects services to monitor their performance against national standards. Some of these standards relate to infection prevention and control and cleanliness. The CQC provides guidance to health and social care providers about meeting their standards, including those for infection prevention and cleanliness in their document *Essential Standards of Quality and Safety.* Outcome 8 under safeguarding and safety contains the relevant information.

WHO Clean Care is Safer Care

This is a World Health Organization initiative, and the goal of Clean Care is Safer Care is to ensure that infection control is acknowledged universally as a solid and essential basis towards patient safety and supports the reduction of healthcare-associated infections and their consequences. It has included a global campaign to improve hand hygiene.

Infection prevention related legislation

The Public Health (Control of Diseases) Act 1984 and Public Health (Infectious Diseases) Regulations 1988

This Act and regulations provide legislation and provisions around such aspects as notifiable diseases and the regulation for control of certain diseases. Under the 1984 Act, any person who knowingly exposes others to an infectious disease is guilty of an offence, either by being infected themselves or by exposing clients to risks from other clients. This includes knowingly exposing others to HIV, for example. Other provisions relate to aspects such as funeral arrangements, port health and exclusion of children from schools and nurseries.

Scenario

You are a nurse working on a paediatric ward and a 7-year-old girl is admitted to your ward with a pyrexia (high temperature) of unknown cause. She has recently returned from a family holiday in India. The medical team that you are working with orders blood and urine tests and it is discovered that she has malaria. Under the Public Health Act, malaria is a notifiable disease so it is required by law to report it to government authorities, and the doctor therefore needs to complete a notification form for this patient under the Act. Such diseases are usually notified by either a doctor or by the laboratory.

The Health and Social Care Act (2008): Code of Practice on the Prevention and Control of Infection and Related Guidance (Department of Health, 2015)

According to the Code of Practice, 'The law states that the Code must be taken into account by the CQC when it makes decisions about registration against the infection prevention requirements 12 (h) and 21 (b). The regulations also say that providers must have regard to the Code when deciding how they will comply with registration requirements' (page 9). The main purposes of this Code are to make the registration requirement for infection prevention clear to all registered providers so that they understand what they need to do to comply; provide guidance for the CQC's staff to make judgement about compliance with the requirements for infection prevention; provide information for people who use the services of a registered provider; provide information for commissioners of services on what they should expect of their providers; and provide information for the general public.

Public health aspects of infection prevention and control

Public health was defined in the Public Health in England report in 1988 as 'the science and art of preventing disease, prolonging life, and promoting health through the organised efforts of society' (Sir Donald Acheson, 1988, page 13). Work in public health is either at a community or population level. According to the Department of Health, 'Public health professionals work with other professional groups to monitor the health status of the community, identify health needs, develop programmes to reduce risk and screen for early disease, control communicable disease, foster policies which promote health, plan and evaluate the provision of healthcare, and manage and implement change.' In relation to infection prevention, the public health function is around communicable disease control. This includes surveillance and detection of communicable diseases, contact tracing and notification relating to infection, outbreak management, promotion of immunisation programmes and **epidemiology**.

Surveillance of communicable diseases and infection is carried out both in the hospital and community settings but in different ways. In hospitals, for example, they may undertake what is known as ALERT organism surveillance where they identify the number of certain infections, such as MRSA **bacteraemias** that occur in their patients over a given time period. Other ALERT organisms include *Clostridium difficile* and other organisms which can cause problems locally, particularly those with some antibiotic resistance. Further information can be found on some of these micro-organisms in Chapter 3. Surveillance programmes may be undertaken so that any changes in the occurrence of infection are identified; to guide action which needs to be taken and to evaluate the effectiveness of interventions put into place such as in infection outbreak situations.

Contact tracing occurs in some infections where people who have been in certain types of contact with an infected individual need to be identified so that further action can be taken. This includes, for example, tracing close contacts of people who have contracted meningococcal disease so that they can be provided with antibiotics in order to prevent secondary cases. Such tracing also occurs in cases of tuberculosis.

A notifiable disease is any disease that is required by law to be reported to government authorities. Each country in the world has a different list of diseases which are notifiable. In England, such diseases are notified by registered medical practitioners (RMPs) to the 'proper officer' at their local council or local health protection team (HPT). They are also required to notify the 'proper officer' of suspected notifiable diseases. All laboratories in England performing a primary diagnostic role must notify Public Health England (PHE) when they confirm a notifiable organism. PHE collects these notifications and publishes analyses of local and national trends every week. The statutory duty to report these diseases is related to the Public Health (Control of Diseases) Act 1984 and the Health Protection (Notification) Regulations 2010.

Activity 1.3	*Evidence-based practice and research*

Go to the government website **www.gov.uk** and find out what the notifiable diseases are in England. Which of these are you aware of?

No answer is provided for this activity as the answers are on the above website.

As you will have found from this activity, there are many diseases which are notifiable. Some of these can cause outbreaks of infection.

Outbreak management is an important public health function and involves the formation of an outbreak team to investigate and control the outbreak. This can occur where an outbreak has been identified either in a hospital or a community-based setting such as a school or related to a setting such as a farm visitor centre or food establishment. Nurses are part of the outbreak management team as are doctors and environmental health professionals.

Scenario

You are working with a school nurse and go to visit a school where the head teacher approaches you for advice as seven students in the same class have developed symptoms of diarrhoea and vomiting. Under the UK definition, this constitutes a possible outbreak and an outbreak management team needs to be organised with the community based staff in your area who manage these outbreaks. This might include the public health or health protection nurse in your area, a consultant in communicable disease control and an environmental health officer. The team will investigate the outbreak to try to identify the cause and prevent further spread if it is caused by an infection.

Immunisation programmes are an important way of minimising the risk of many infections. Programmes in the UK begin in childhood (such as the MMR) and continue throughout life onto the elderly population (such as the flu jab). Nurses involved in such programmes include school nurses, health visitors, practice nurses, district nurses and those working in nursing homes. Nurses therefore fulfil a vital role in immunisation against infectious disease.

Epidemiology is concerned with the diagnosis and treatment of disease (not just infection) at a population level. This differs from the work of a GP, for example, who considers patients individually. Epidemiology contributes to public health policy worldwide and is important in the prevention of disease. When considering infection, epidemiologists believe that most diseases have more than one cause. This might relate to the organisms causing the infection, how at risk a patient is and how the environment that the patient is in contributes. These factors are considered further in the chain of infection in Chapter 2.

Activity 1.4   *Multiple choice questions*

1. What is the reported prevalence of HCAI in England?

    a) 6.4%
    b) 7.4%
    c) 8.4%
    d) 9.0%
    e) 10%

2. What proportion of HCAIs are considered to be avoidable?

    a) 5–20%
    b) 10–25%

c) 15–30%
d) 20–35%
e) 25–40%

3. Which organisation leads the Clean Care is Safer Care initiative?

   a) The Department of Health
   b) Public Health England
   c) The Healthcare Infection Society
   d) The World Health Organization
   e) The ECDC

4. Which of the following diseases is not on the list of notifiable diseases in England?

   a) Food poisoning
   b) Malaria
   c) Measles
   d) MRSA
   e) Tuberculosis

Answers are provided at the end of the chapter.

The above activity should have tested your knowledge relating to what we have covered in this chapter to ensure that you have understood what you have read and learned from the previous activities.

Chapter summary

This chapter has introduced you to the scale of the problem of healthcare-associated infection and its consequences to the people involved. It has also considered the organisations available to support nurses in preventing such infections. The public health function is an important one in the investigation, prevention and management of communicable diseases and infection and this chapter has briefly summarised some of the relevant aspects of this function.

Activities and scenarios: Brief outline answers

Activity 1.1: Reflection (page 6)

Consider what occurred at East Maidstone and Tunbridge Wells Trust in relation to an outbreak of *Clostridium difficile* by searching online. What do you think the consequences have been of this outbreak to this NHS Trust?

Your answer should have mentioned issues such as public reputation and patient confidence in their local hospital. The media was involved in heavy reporting on this organisation which had consequences for other hospitals.

Activity 1.2: Critical thinking (page 7)

Consider the case study above. What are the possible effects of this infection on Julian, the hospital staff and the hospital as an organisation?

Your answer should have considered consequences to Julian in terms of a longer stay in hospital and loss of earnings as he is self-employed. There may also be prescription costs on discharge from hospital. In terms of staff, you might have thought about how staff feel when one of their patients acquires an infection in hospital and about any investigation that might be warranted by this incidence of infection. For the organisation, there might be consequences related to targets for some infections and publication of data about rates of infection.

Activity 1.4: MCQs (pages 12–13)

1. What is the reported prevalence of HCAI in England?

    a) 6.4%

2. What proportion of HCAIs are considered to be avoidable?

    c) 15–30%

3. Which organisation leads the Clean Care is Safer Care initiative?

    d) The World Health Organization

4. Which of the following diseases is not on the list of notifiable diseases in England?

    d) MRSA

Further reading

Department of Health (2015) *The Health and Social Care Act (2008): Code of Practice on the Prevention and Control of Infection and Related Guidance.* London: DH.

This document is a useful resource for students in understanding the national requirements for health and social care providers relating to cleanliness and infection control.

Useful websites

www.ips.uk.net (The Infection Prevention Society)

This site has aspects for both members and non-members and has links to audit and quality improvement tools.

www.his.org.uk (The Healthcare Infection Society)

This site provides documents such as the epic3 guidelines and other infection related documents which can be accessed by anyone.

www.ecdc.europa.eu (The ECDC)

The ECDC website provides freely available publications, data and tools and news updates from across Europe.

www.england.nhs.uk (NHS England)

The National Patient Safety Agency information now appears on this website and the organisation now leads and contributes to improved, safe patient care by informing, supporting and influencing the health sector and this site provides reporting mechanisms for incidents.

www.cqc.org.uk (The Care Quality Commission)

This site provides information for both professionals and the public about the required national standards, how these can be met and how organisations which have been inspected have been rated.

www.gov.uk/government/collections/immunisation

Immunisation against infectious disease, known as The Green Book.

This website contains valuable information about the immunisation schedule within the UK and about the illnesses that are vaccine preventable. This is regularly updated when immunisation schedules change so it is worthwhile keeping this as a favourite.

www.gov.uk/government/organisations/public-health-england

This is the Public Health England website which provides updated information on infection.

www.publichealthwales.wales.nhs.uk

This is the Public Health Wales website and it provides information in both Welsh and English and a link to the Welsh infection prevention and control policies.

www.publichealth.hscni.net

This is the website for the Public Health Agency in Northern Ireland.

www.hps.scot.nhs.uk

This is the website for Health Protection Scotland and it provides a link to the Scottish national infection prevention and control manual.

http://infectioncontrolmanual.co.ni

This link leads to the Northern Ireland infection prevention and control manual.

Chapter 2
Introduction to microbiology

NMC Standards for Pre-registration Nursing Education

This chapter will address the following competencies:

Domain 3: Nursing practice and decision-making

Generic competencies
2. All nurses must possess a broad knowledge of the structure and functions of the human body, and other relevant knowledge from the life, behavioural and social sciences as applied to health, ill health, disability, ageing and death. They must have an in-depth knowledge of common physical and mental health problems and treatments in their own field of practice, including co-morbidity and physiological and psychological vulnerability.
7. All nurses must be able to recognise and interpret signs of normal and deteriorating mental and physical health and respond promptly to maintain or improve the health and comfort of the service user, acting to keep them and others safe.

NMC Essential Skills Clusters: Infection Control

This chapter will address the following ESCs:

* Participates in assessing and planning care appropriate to the risk of infection thus promoting the safety of service users (Progression point 2).
* Recognises potential signs of infection and reports them to a relevant senior member of staff (Progression point 2).
* Acts to address potential risks within a timely manner including in the home setting (Progression point 2).
* Applies knowledge of transmission routes in describing, recognising and reporting situations where there is a need for standard infection control precautions (Progression point 2).
* Recognises infection risks and reports and acts in situations where there is a need for health promotion and protection and public health strategies (Progression point 3).
* Initiates and maintains appropriate measures to prevent and control infection according to routes of transmission of organism, in order to protect service users, members of the public and other staff (Progression point 3).

Introduction

Microbiology forms the basis for our actions in infection prevention and control and therefore how we care for our patients as nurses, whatever field of nursing we are studying or working in. From the previous chapter you should now understand the costs to both healthcare services and patients of both infection and healthcare-associated infection and therefore be aware of the importance of sound knowledge and good practice in order to prevent all avoidable infections. A knowledge of microbiology will enable you to consider the rationale for care that you provide and to provide explanations to your patients about what is happening to them.

This chapter begins by considering what microbiology is and why nurses need to study it. It then goes on to look at the significance of normal flora and what the sources of infection are. After discussing the chain of infection and its six links there follows information about the routes of transmission of infection as one of the links in the chain and then consideration of the signs and symptoms that patients with infection might present with. Another link in the chain of infection is then discussed in terms of risk factors for infection that identify someone as a susceptible host. Finally, there is an overview of the process of infection and virulence factors which enable pathogens to evade a person's immune system. Throughout the chapter are activities for you to complete which will enable you to link the theory of microbiology to practice.

Case study

Ethel is a 72-year-old patient who lives alone with her dog and cat and is seen by her local practice nurse complaining of a painful cut on her leg. On seeing the patient, the nurse asks her about symptoms that she has other than the pain and examines the cut herself. From her knowledge of signs and symptoms of infection, she suspects that the cut may be infected and obtains a wound swab to send to the laboratory so that any organism present can be identified. This is based on Ethel's pain, redness around the cut and oozing from the cut. She applies a dressing to the cut then talks to Ethel about where she may have got the infection from, how it might be transmitted to others and how Ethel can stop this happening. She also identifies what factors increase Ethel's risk of infection and whether any of these can be addressed.

The practice nurse is able to do these things because of her knowledge of microbiology.

Microbiology

This is the study of microscopic organisms, that is, those which cannot be seen with the naked eye (Ford, 2014). In healthcare, such organisms are divided into the following groups which are discussed in Chapters 3–5:

- Bacteria
- Viruses
- Fungi
- Parasites including protozoa
- Prions

Micro-organisms exist everywhere, including on and inside the human body and in the environment but not all of them are capable of causing infection. Even those that are capable can be present on or within people, multiplying, without causing any tissue reaction, any symptoms or any disease – this is known as colonisation. Infection occurs when organisms invade a body site and multiply, causing a reaction in the tissues, symptoms and disease.

Why do nurses need to know about microbiology?

There are several reasons why a level of knowledge about microbiology is essential for nursing practice. First, some of the organisms that live on or in our body have the potential to cause infection and the prevention of infection in both ourselves and our patients is an important aspect of nursing care. Some micro-organisms can cause infectious diseases and nurses need to be aware of how to protect themselves, their patients, visitors and other members of staff from these and how to minimise the risk of spread. Nurses also need to be able to explain about infection, its causes, its transmission and its prevention and treatment to their patients. It is worth noting that microbiology underpins infection prevention and control processes, so in order to understand fully the need for these processes we also need to understand their microbiological basis. Microbiological knowledge is also part of the NMCs Essential Skills Clusters (NMC, 2010) and is therefore a required element of both progression through your degree programme and of registering as a nurse with the NMC at the end of your programme.

Human flora

Some organisms live in or on the body but cause no harm – these are referred to as **commensals** or human normal **flora**. Table 2.1 identifies the normal flora found in different areas of the body. While these organisms cause no harm in these sites, if they are transferred to other sites in the body they have the potential to cause infection.

Normal flora has a range of functions within the body. Such flora can prevent other pathogenic bacteria from multiplying and causing infection by both competing for nutrients and by taking up space. In the gut normal flora aids digestion and produces essential vitamins. Stimulation is provided by normal flora to produce low level antibodies which can act against infection. It therefore has a role to play in immunity against disease.

Site	Normal flora
Skin	*Staphylococcus epidermidis* Micrococci Diphtheroids *Corynebacterium* Enteric bacilli *Propioniumbacterium acnes*
Oropharynx	*Streptococcus viridans* Diphtheroids *Moraxella catarrhalis* *Corynebacterium* *Haemophilus* Spirochetes
Large intestine	*Bacteroides* *Escherichia coli* *Streptococcus faecalis* Proteus Clostridia Lactobacilli Enteric bacilli
Vagina	Lactobacilli *Staphylococcus epidermidis* Streptococcus *Bacteroides* *Mycoplasma*
Central nervous system Bladder and urinary tract Lower respiratory tract	All normally sterile so no normal flora

Table 2.1: Normal flora

(Harvey et al., 2007)

Normal flora is generally considered to be the micro-organisms which are frequently found on or inside the bodies of healthy people. In addition to the organisms identified within the table, some people have flora which others do not. If an organism is found in more than 5% of the population it can be considered to be normal flora, despite the fact that more than 90% of the population do not carry it. Such organisms do not usually cause infection in the carriers but may cause infection in other people who are not carriers if it is transferred to them. An example of this is that around 10% of the population carry the meningococcus bacterium in their respiratory tract. This would be considered to be normal flora in this 10% of people but not in the other 90% of the population. Similarly, around 10% of people are carriers of group A streptococcus worldwide (see Chapter 3) in their nose and throat and this is therefore normal flora in this 10% (Abdissa et al., 2011; Prajapati et al., 2012).

Normal flora is not harmful in its normal habitat. As has been identified, however, it can cause infection such as urinary tract infections being caused by colonic flora and surgical site infections by skin flora. Antibiotics can also alter **indigenous** flora which naturally occurs at certain body sites by acting against it. These antibiotics can kill bacteria which is considered to be healthy and which are necessary in the body and this allows other flora including other bacteria or fungi to proliferate or multiply causing infection. This can result in diarrhoea and candidiasis, for example.

In terms of establishing normal flora on the human body, this commences once the foetal membranes are ruptured prior to a baby being born. Within a few hours of birth, the baby is colonised with micro-organisms from the mother's vagina, skin and respiratory tract. Within 6–12 hours after birth, the infant's colon is colonised. It is clear, then, that normal flora is established very early in life.

Some flora is termed **transient** – these are micro-organisms that are temporarily present and are those which cause most issues in the healthcare setting. For example, a member of staff may touch an environmental surface and pick up micro-organisms on the hands. If they then touch a patient, these micro-organisms may be transferred from their hands onto the patient – the micro-organisms are then no longer on the hands of the healthcare worker. Such flora has significance when we discuss standard precautions, and in particular hand hygiene, in a later chapter.

Pathogens are those micro-organisms which cause disease, and in this case infection, and are sometimes referred to as **virulent** strains as opposed to non-virulent strains of an organism which are not considered to be pathogenic and do not cause disease. Pathogens can be divided into three main groups: conventional pathogens, which are not part of the human normal flora so MRSA might be an example; conditional, which cause infection in certain conditions, such as *Escherichia coli* (*E. coli*) when it is in the bladder rather than in the gut; and opportunistic pathogens which thrive when a specific opportunity arises, such as *Candida albicans*, when other flora is diminished, such as in antibiotic use. Opportunistic pathogens also cause problems in patients who are immuno-compromised as they take advantage of the person's diminished capacity to fight infection.

When exposed to pathogens, not all people develop an infection or become ill. This is for several reasons. Sometimes the pathogen comes into contact with a body site where it cannot multiply due to, for example, a lack of favourable conditions in that site for that particular pathogen to grow. Also, if at that body site there are not the specific receptors which some pathogens need to cause infection, the pathogens will be unable to cause infection. In some body sites there are antibacterial properties which can stop multiplication of bacteria or even destroy them – this might include enzymes or some normal flora; normal flora can also inhibit pathogen multiplication by using up nutrients that the pathogens might require. The person's susceptibility or immunity to specific infections also play a role and often the immune system will destroy pathogens before they are able to multiply.

Sources of infection

Normal flora is important when we consider sources of infection. These can be considered to be endogenous or exogenous. **Endogenous** sources of infection are those seen as coming from within.

These could therefore be considered as self-infections. These can occur if patients move flora around their bodies to sites where they are no longer normal, causing infections in themselves (Haas et al., 2005). An example of this could be an *E. coli* urinary tract infection. *E. coli*, particularly in women, can be transferred from the bowel to the bladder due to the short urethra in women, causing an infection. This is why women are encouraged to wipe front to back as opposed to back to front after going to the toilet. Another example might be someone who moves some of their flora into a surgical wound on their hands – if this occurs within a specified time after surgery it would be considered as healthcare-associated, despite being transmitted by the patient themselves.

Clearly some infections are transmitted from elsewhere – in the healthcare setting this might be from other people or the environment and in other areas it might be pets or other animals, for example. These are of an **exogenous** source. The majority of healthcare-associated infections acquired exogenously are caused by transfer on staff hands. They might also be acquired through dust and skin scales in the environment, as an example, which some micro-organisms use as a reservoir (see Figure 2.1) (Greenwood et al., 2012).

Case study

Consider Sheila, a 43-year-old woman who is one of the 10% of people who have group A streptococcus as part of their normal flora on their oropharynx (one of the parts of the throat). One day, while chopping vegetables, she cut her finger. She then proceeded to do what many people would. She put her cut finger into her mouth. At this stage she transmitted what was normal flora into her bloodstream where it was no longer normal and this may have resulted in the septicaemia for which she was treated in intensive care. This is a prime example of an infection from an endogenous source as it is highly likely that she did not 'catch' the infection from someone else, but that it was caused by transmitting an organism from a normal site to a site where it was not normal. Moving normal flora from one area of the body to another can therefore be a significant source of infection and can have serious consequences in some cases.

Various body fluids, excretions and secretions can act as a source of infection, beyond what many would consider to be obvious sources. Some of these include:

- Blood
- Urine
- Faeces
- Vomit
- Sputum
- Skin scales
- Pericardial fluid
- Synovial fluid
- Breast milk
- Ear wax

- Vaginal secretions
- Semen
- Pus
- Wound exudate

The chain of infection

The chain of infection has six links which represent the events which must occur in order for an infection to happen. Without one of the links in the chain, infection will not occur. This can therefore assist nurses and other healthcare professions in the prevention and control of infection as in practice we can remove one of the links.

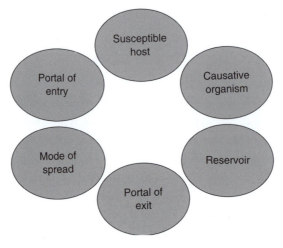

Figure 2.1: The chain of infection

- *Causative organism* – this might be a virus, bacterium, fungus, parasite or prion, in other words a micro-organism which is capable of causing an infection.
- *Reservoir* – different organisms have different reservoirs where they may live and multiply without causing harm. These reservoirs can include people, animals, food, plants, dust and skin scales. MRSA, for example, can use dust and skin scales in the environment as a reservoir in which it can live so this would include the hospital environment.
- *Portal of exit* – this is the way that a micro-organism exits from the reservoir. This might be in a secretion or excretion for example.
- *Mode of spread/route of transmission* – this is the means by which the organism travels from the reservoir to the person. The four main routes of transmission are covered below.
- *Portal of entry* – this is the way in which the micro-organism enters the body. This might be through the digestive system, the respiratory tract or the bloodstream, for example.
- *Susceptible host* – this is the person at risk of infection. Factors which increase the risk of infection are discussed later.

In order to interrupt the chain of infection, in infection prevention and control we might interrupt the mode of spread by hand hygiene, as an example, or remove the reservoir by cleaning the environment of dust and skin scales. We can also reduce susceptibility to some infections in the host by immunisation. The next activity will prompt you to relate this to what you have already experienced in practice or it is something to consider when you are out in practice.

Activity 2.1   *Reflection*

Consider a patient with an infection who you have cared for. In order to prevent the spread of this infection to others, think about what links in the chain of infection you addressed as a nurse. If you have not yet been out in practice, undertake this activity during your first placement.

Suggested points to consider can be found at the end of this chapter.

One of the links in the chain of infection that you might have considered in the activity above is the mode of spread/route of transmission which we will now look at further.

Routes of transmission of infection

There are four main routes of transmission or modes of spread of infection. Some micro-organisms have more than one mode of spread.

a) The airborne route – this includes spread by aerosols and droplets in the air or through contact with respiratory secretions. Examples of organisms spread by this route include pulmonary tuberculosis and influenza.

b) The contact route – this can be direct or indirect contact. Direct is person-to-person transmission where infections are transferred by direct personal contact between individuals. This also includes microbes transferred by touch on the hands of healthcare workers, for example. Indirect might be via food, water and inanimate objects such as patient equipment. Examples of organisms transmitted by this route include MRSA, scabies and headlice.

c) The faecal–oral route – microbes spread by this route generally cause gastro-intestinal infections as such microbes are ingested via contaminated food or drink. The spread may be via contaminated hands such as during food preparation, via food and water contaminated with organisms and via inanimate objects such as kitchen utensils. Examples of organisms transmitted by this route include *Salmonella enteritidis*, *Campylobacter jejuni* and hepatitis A.

d) The blood and body fluid route – this can be considered horizontal or vertical. Horizontal transmission might occur through accidental inoculation, contamination of damaged skin such as a wound, contamination of mucous membranes such as the eyes or through sexual transmission. Vertical transmission is when a foetus is in-utero or during delivery. Examples of organisms transmitted by this route include hepatitis B and C, HIV and malaria.

It is important in practice that you are aware of the routes of transmission of the infections that you may be exposed to – the next activity will enable you to consider this.

Activity 2.2   *Evidence-based practice and research*

What are the main routes of transmission of the following micro-organisms? Some may have more than one route. Possible sources of information to assist you with this activity include the Public Health England website whose address is provided at the end of the previous chapter.

a) Chicken pox
b) Pulmonary tuberculosis
c) Hepatitis E
d) Measles
e) Legionnaire's disease
f) Influenza
g) Threadworms
h) Ringworm

Answers can be found at the end of the chapter.

Now that you have considered the routes of transmission of infection, we now need to look at how infection is identified in our patients in cases where we may have been unable to interrupt the transmission routes.

Signs and symptoms of infection

Patient scenario

Imagine you are a nurse working on a surgical ward. You are caring for patients before and after surgery and therefore need to be aware of the complications related to surgery so that you can effectively care for these patients post-operatively. Carl is a 28-year-old who has recently had a hernia repair and he complains that he is feeling unwell two days after his operation. You undertake his usual observations and find that he is pyrexial at 38.5 °C – his pulse, blood pressure and respiratory rate are within normal limits. At this stage your role would be to consider the causes of pyrexia and to investigate further what other symptoms Carl has so that you can better manage his treatment and care. One of the possible causes of pyrexia is infection – you therefore need to be aware of other signs and symptoms of infection so that you can identify these in Carl in order to take further action.

In order to identify whether the patient has an infection, signs and symptoms need to be considered. This is because the presence of an organism does not necessarily indicate infection; it may instead be colonisation. Infection diagnosis therefore combines signs and symptoms of infection with the presence of an organism. There are some general signs and symptoms which may indicate infection and if these are present, further investigation is needed to identify the site and cause of the infection. Not all signs and symptoms will always be present and effective identification of indications of infection comes with clinical experience. In nursing, the words 'signs' and 'symptoms' are used interchangeably but in microbiological terms they have distinct differences – it is therefore worth noting these here so that you are aware of this when reading other microbiology textbooks. A **symptom** is considered to be something that the patient experiences and is therefore considered to be subjective which means that it is not easily measured by others – this includes things such as pain, nausea or dizziness. A **sign** is more objective and is therefore measurable by others so might include an abnormal heart rate, a high temperature, changes in blood pressure or a raised white cell count – all these can be recorded and measured objectively.

General signs and symptoms of infection might include **pyrexia**, **inflammation**, pain, pus production, **tachycardia**, confusion in the elderly and a raised white cell count. As a nurse it is important to understand why these symptoms occur so that infection can be identified appropriately and explanations can be provided to patients about their condition.

Pyrexia is a normal body response to infection and is thought to strengthen the immune response. Pyrexia does not always indicate infection, but if someone has a pyrexia of unknown origin, infection should be one of the possibilities considered – in order to confirm this, other signs and symptoms should be sought to gain a clearer picture of the patient's condition.

Inflammation is a protective mechanism within the body which, in infection, aims to remove the invading pathogen and initiate the repair process. It involves the cells of the host, blood vessels and proteins and is how vascular tissues respond to the invading pathogens.

Pain is often a consequence of inflammation and is a normal symptom in some infections.

Nausea and vomiting are thought to be caused by the endotoxins which are released when invading micro-organisms are **lysed** or broken down as part of the body's immune response to infection.

Pus production occurs as a result of the immune response when white blood cells are sent to the site of infection. Pus is a thick discharge which consists of white blood cells, damaged cells and dead tissue. It can vary in colour from white through to yellow and green and can be blood-stained.

Tachycardia can occur as a consequence of pyrexia in infection.

A raised white cell count in a blood test is evidence of the immune response as white cell production is increased as a response to invasion by an infectious agent. However, changes in white cell count can also be an indication of other conditions besides infection, so a raised white cell count alone is not definitive proof of infection.

As well as being aware of the general signs and symptoms of infection, as nurses we need to be aware of specific symptoms which relate to infections in different areas of the body. The next activity will enable you to consider this.

Activity 2.3   *Evidence-based practice and research*

For the following sites, identify what the signs and symptoms might be:

a) Eye infection

b Urinary tract infection

c) Wound infection

d) Chest infection

Answers can be found at the end of the chapter.

We have so far considered the route of transmission link in the chain of infection and the signs and symptoms that patients may demonstrate when they have an infection. Another link that we now need to look at is the susceptible host so that we can identify patients who are at higher risk of infection and act to reduce risks wherever possible.

Risk factors for infection: the susceptible host

There are many factors which increase a patient's risk of infection, some of which we can address and others which we cannot change – in infection prevention we aim to minimise risk as far as possible, but this still means that some patients remain at high risk of infection. Some of these factors are specific to the patient and others are related to the environment in which they are being cared for such as a hospital, a nursing or residential home, a clinic or GP surgery, a special needs school or the patient's own home.

Patient-specific risk factors for infection include:

- Age – increasing age and the young

- Chronic disease, e.g. diabetes

- Psychological wellbeing

- Nutritional status, e.g. having the right vitamins and minerals within the diet to maintain a healthy immune system

- Medication, e.g. steroids

- Medical intervention such as surgery

- Lifestyle factors, e.g. smoking

- Job, e.g. being a healthcare worker can increase the risk of infection with organisms such as *Clostridium difficile*

- The presence of a wound
- The presence of an invasive device, e.g. a urinary catheter.

There may also be risk factors associated with where a patient is being cared for. These might include factors such as:

- Overcrowding
- Sharing patient equipment
- Mass catering such as in nursing and residential homes
- Non-compliance issues among staff
- Contact with patients with infections
- Lack of appropriate facilities for clinical practice, such as in some patients' homes.

It is important that patients at high risk of infection are identified and that appropriate precautions are put into place. These precautions are discussed in later chapters. In many healthcare organisations, risk assessment tools will be used on patient admission to identify those at particular risk but these vary from a simple one question assessment to a tool which may cover several pages.

Activity 2.4   *Reflection*

Think about the placements you have had so far. What infection risk assessment tools have been used? How useful were they in deciding what nursing interventions to put into place for individual patients?

Suggested points can be found at the end of this chapter.

So far we have looked at how infection is transmitted, what signs and symptoms might indicate infection and what factors increase risk of infection. We will now consider the process of infection and how this might link to the signs and symptoms that patients experience.

The infection process

Depending on which textbook you read, the infection process will be divided differently with numerous stages. In order to assist you to understand this, this book will consider the process in two ways: steps in pathogenesis of infection and phases in the course of an infection. The first considers the sequence of events from entry of the pathogen into the body to damage of the cells within the patient. The second looks at the phases which occur once the pathogen has entered the body, from pathogen arrival to recovery of the patient. It is important to consider these stages in these two ways as the latter considers what symptoms the patient experiences at each stage or phase which is important in nursing care whereas the former is more concerned with the mechanisms involved in the development of infection in terms of microbiology and immunology.

Steps in the pathogenesis of infection or infectious disease

The first stage is entry of the pathogen into the body via one of the portals of entry as mentioned when we discussed the chain of infection. The pathogen then attaches itself to some tissue or tissues within the body – as explained earlier this may be in an inappropriate site where the next step of multiplication cannot occur. If the pathogen is able to multiply, it can do this at one body site causing a more localised infection or may multiply in multiple sites around the body, leading to a more systemic infection. Following multiplication of the pathogen, there is invasion or spread. Following this the pathogen will go on to evade the immune defences mounted by the body and will then continue to cause damage to body tissues – this can be so severe that it causes death. It is therefore important that we recognise the signs and symptoms of infection and that we act quickly to treat infection in order to minimise the risk of severe disease. The aspects of pathogens which allow them to evade the body's immune defences in order to cause tissue damage are discussed later.

Phases in the course of an infection or infectious disease

There are generally considered to be four phases once a pathogen has entered the body. *The incubation phase* is the time period between the entry of the pathogen and symptoms beginning. There are therefore no symptoms for the patient during this phase. Incubation periods differ from one pathogen to another and may vary from hours to months. The incubation periods of some common pathogens are shown in Table 2.2. Following incubation comes *the prodromal phase* which is the time when patients start to feel as if they might be developing an illness but not yet feeling any of the actual symptoms of infection. For example, they may feel a little more tired than usual. During the phase of *illness* the patient experiences the symptoms of infection. Generally infectious diseases are most transmissible during this phase. Following illness is a phase of *convalescence* during which the patient recovers. This can be quite long in some infections, for example glandular fever which involves infection with the Epstein Barr virus. It needs to be identified here that while the infection is no longer considered to be active, it may have caused permanent tissue damage to the patient. This may include damage to areas such as the brain in meningitis related infections.

Some infections seem to lie outside of the normal phases of infectious disease. For example, *latent infections* are those which move from being symptomatic to showing no symptoms (being asymptomatic) then going back to symptomatic. Infections which may demonstrate latency include cold sores, genital herpes and shingles (all herpes viruses) and syphilis (caused by the bacterium *Treponema pallidum*). For example, in the case of cold sores which are caused by herpes simplex virus, patients do not have any symptoms when they first become infected. The virus lays dormant within the body and then every so often the virus can be activated by certain triggers which might include menstruation in women or fatigue. This may happen several times per year in some patients whereas in others, though they have the virus, they never have any symptoms.

The body mounts an immune response to infection which can cause some of the symptoms associated with it – it is therefore not only infection which causes symptoms but also the body's response to it. The immune response is divided into specific and non-specific systems. It is not within the remit of this book to discuss immunity and the immune system – further information on this can be gained from anatomy and physiology texts (example textbooks can be found under further reading at the end of this chapter).

Pathogen	Incubation period
Chicken pox	1–3 weeks
Diphtheria	2–5 days
Hepatitis A	15–45 days
Hepatitis B	30–180 days
Influenza	1–3 days
Measles	10–12 days
Mumps	12–25 days
Norovirus	1–3 days
Pertussis	Up to 21 days
Rubella	14–21 days
Tetanus	4–21 days

Table 2.2: Example incubation periods

(Public Health England 2013a)

Virulence factors

These are the aspects of pathogens which allow them to evade the patient's immune defences and therefore cause damage in that patient's tissues. This book provides a brief overview of these, but more detailed information about virulence factors can be found in the Burton textbook (see further reading at the end of this chapter) for those students with a special interest in this aspect of infection.

Pathogens have specific types of cells that they are able to attach themselves to within the body – if these cells are not present then the pathogen cannot cause infection. This is why some pathogens infect humans but not animals and some infect some sites within the body but not others – this was referred to earlier when considering why sometimes people are exposed to pathogens but do not become infected.

In Chapter 3 we will consider the structure of bacteria but for the purposes of this section you need to understand that some bacteria are surrounded by *capsules* and others are not. Those that have capsules cannot be engulfed by cells called **phagocytes** which are part of the immune response. This means that they cannot be destroyed by these cells – bacterial capsules are therefore considered to be a virulence factor. *Flagella* are also part of some bacteria and these allow some bacteria to reach areas of the body which those without flagella cannot reach – they also enable these bacteria to move more quickly to avoid being engulfed by phagocytes.

Some pathogens produce exoenzymes that enable them to evade the host's defences which means that they can invade or cause damage to a person's tissues. These include necrotising enzymes which destroy tissues and **coagulase** which can form a coat of **fibrin** to protect the pathogen from host defences. They also include **kinases** which enable pathogens to escape from clots and hyaluronidase which can enable pathogens to spread through connective tissue. Collagenase enables pathogens to invade tissues by breaking down collagen and haemolysins cause damage to red blood cells, while lecithinase can destroy cell membranes.

Some pathogens can produce *toxins* which are considered to be poisonous substances. Endotoxins are a part of the cell wall of Gram-negative bacteria (see Chapter 3) and can cause septicaemia and shock. Exotoxins are secreted by some pathogens and include neurotoxins which affect the central nervous system, enterotoxins which affect the gastro-intestinal tract, exfoliative toxins which affect the skin and leucocidins which destroy white blood cells.

Pathogens also have mechanisms by which they can escape the body's immune responses. Some pathogens, for example, periodically change their surfaces so that this interferes with antibody production. Other pathogens can camouflage themselves by coating themselves with body proteins. Some pathogens also produce enzymes which destroy some antibodies.

Some special circumstances in infection

While there are a range of responses to infection within the body, it is important to have some knowledge and understanding of some of the extreme consequences. We will now therefore consider two.

Necrotising fasciitis

Also called the 'flesh eating disease', this is a bacterial infection that affects the soft tissue and **fascia**. It can occur following a cut or some other opportunity for the bacteria to enter the body, such as surgery. Public Health England (2013b) identifies specific symptoms which present themselves at different stages as follows:

Early symptoms (usually within 24 hours) include:

- intense and severe pain which may seem out of proportion to any external signs of infection on the skin;
- a small but painful cut or scratch on the skin;
- fever and other flu-like symptoms.

Advanced symptoms (usually within 3 to 4 days) include:

- swelling of the painful area, accompanied by a rash;
- diarrhoea and vomiting;
- large dark blotches, that will turn into blisters and fill up with fluid.

Critical symptoms (usually within 4 to 5 days) include:

- severe fall in blood pressure;
- toxic shock from the poisons released by the bacteria;
- unconsciousness as the body weakens.

Though the condition can be caused by various bacteria, the main cause is *Streptococcus pyogenes* (see Chapter 3). It is treated with antibiotics and some patients may require surgery to remove the affected area which may, in some cases, be a limb.

Sepsis and related conditions

Sepsis occurs when there is an inflammatory response in the whole body to an infection, instead of just at the site of infection. You may also hear the terms septicaemia or blood poisoning, though these are not strictly the same as sepsis. It usually occurs as a result of infection with bacteria but can also occur with viruses, fungi and parasites. Septicaemia refers to illness which is the result of the uncontrolled spread of either bacteria or toxins produced by bacteria throughout the bloodstream. Septicaemia is therefore considered under the umbrella term 'sepsis' but not all sepsis is septicaemia.

Sepsis is defined by Dellinger et al. (2012) as the presence of infection together with systemic manifestations of infection. There are specific criteria which need to be met for a diagnosis of sepsis which include a temperature above 38.3°C or below 36°C, a heart rate of above 90 bpm, a blood sugar of above 7.7 mmol/L in the absence of diabetes, plus other inflammatory, **haemodynamic**, organ dysfunction and tissue perfusion variables (further information on these can be found at the website given at the end of this chapter). Severe sepsis is considered to have occurred when, in addition to sepsis, there is either sepsis-induced organ dysfunction or tissue **hypoperfusion**. Septic shock occurs in severe sepsis when there is cardiovascular dysfunction. This is usually indicated by low blood pressure which does not improve when fluids are given. Clearly, then, sepsis can result in death.

In 2015 the Surviving Sepsis Campaign updated their previous management bundle and the most recent guidelines provide actions which must be taken within three hours and six hours.

Within three hours of the patient presenting with sepsis, we should:

1. Measure lactate level.
2. Obtain blood cultures prior to administration of antibiotics.
3. Administer broad spectrum antibiotics.
4. Administer 3 mL/kg crystalloid for hypotension or lactate ≥4 mmol/L.

Within six hours, we should:

5. Apply vasopressors (for hypotension that does not respond to initial fluid resuscitation) to maintain a mean arterial pressure (MAP) ≥6 mmHg.

6. In the event of persistent hypotension after initial fluid administration (MAP <6 mmHg) or if initial lactate was ≥4 mmol/L, re-assess volume status and tissue perfusion and document findings.

7. Re-measure lactate if initial lactate elevated.

These issues might seem quite complicated at this stage, but you need not worry as sepsis management has set protocols within healthcare organisations which qualified healthcare professionals follow and which you can therefore learn from should a case arise while you are in placement.

It is now time to review what you have learned within this chapter by undertaking some multiple choice questions.

Activity 2.5   *Multiple choice questions*

1. Which of the following is NOT a link in the chain of infection?

   a) Reservoir
   b) Mode of spread
   c) Portal of exit
   d) Decontamination
   e) Susceptible host

2. Which of the following are possible signs and symptoms of a wound infection?

   a) Productive cough, pyrexia, chest pain
   b) Confusion, pyrexia, pain on urination
   c) Exudate, redness, pain
   d) Genital warts, pain on intercourse, pyrexia
   e) Sticky eye, itching, pyrexia

3. Which of the following micro-organisms is considered to be part of the normal flora of the skin?

   a) *Staphylococcus epidermidis*
   b) *Haemophilus*
   c) Lactobacilli
   d) *Proteus*
   e) Clostridia

4. What is the main route of transmission of MRSA?

   a) Airborne
   b) Blood-borne – vertical
   c) Blood-borne – horizontal
   d) Contact
   e) Faecal–oral

5. Which of the following sites is normally sterile?

   a) The skin
   b) The colon
   c) The vagina
   d) The bladder
   e) The oropharynx

6. Which of the following is NOT a virulence factor?

   a) A phagocyte
   b) Flagella
   c) Exoenzymes
   d) Toxins
   e) Bacterial capsules

Answers are provided at the end of the chapter.

Chapter summary

This chapter has introduced you to the topic of microbiology and has explained why nurses need such knowledge. By considering issues such as the chain of infection, routes of transmission of infection and risk factors for infection, we have been able to relate microbiology to the care of our patients and gained an understanding so that we can explain transmission and risks to patients. You should also now be able to consider more clearly the signs and symptoms of infection which your patients may present with so that you can recognise potential signs and act quickly to manage the patient appropriately.

Activities: Brief outline answers

Activity 2.1: Reflection (page 23)

Consider a patient that you have cared for with an infection. In order to prevent the spread of this infection to others, think about what links in the chain of infection you addressed as a nurse.

Issues you should have considered here should have been related to the six links in the chain of infection. For example you might have considered a patient with a specific infection and thought about the route of transmission of that infection, what risk factors your patient had for infection, what the possible reservoir was for the micro-organism which caused the infection and how the organism might leave the patient and enter another person.

Activity 2.2: Evidence-based practice and research (page 24)

What are the main routes of transmission of the following micro-organisms? Some may have more than one route.

a) Chicken pox: Airborne and contact
b) Pulmonary tuberculosis: Airborne

c) Hepatitis E: Faecal–oral
d) Measles: Airborne and contact
e) Legionnaire's disease: Airborne
f) Influenza: Airborne
g) Threadworms: Faecal–oral
h) Ringworm: Contact

Activity 2.3: Evidence-based practice and research (page 26)

For the following sites, identify what the signs and symptoms might be:

a) – Eye infection – symptoms might include redness, swelling, pain, itching, an increase in tear production and a sticky eye.

b) – Urinary tract infection – symptoms might include pain on passing urine, frequency, urgency, blood in urine, cloudy urine, offensive smelling urine, pyrexia, confusion in the elderly, incontinence.

c) – Wound infection – symptoms might include pain, redness, heat, wound exudate, pyrexia, offensive smell.

d) – Chest infection – symptoms might include a cough, back or chest pain, dyspnoea, sputum production and blue lips.

Activity 2.4: Reflection (page 27)

Think about the placements you have had so far. What infection risk assessment tools have been used? How useful were they in deciding what nursing interventions to put into place for individual patients?

Possible tools that you might have been exposed to include the Kettering Infection Predictor, the tool published by Capita's journal *The Risk Resource* or other locally produced tools. You might also have been exposed to risk assessment which only includes one question which relates to a specific infection such as, 'Has the patient previously tested positive for MRSA, *Clostridium difficile* or CPE?' Some of these you will have found more useful than others in advising you about the care of individual patients.

Activity 2.5: MCQs (pages 32–3)

1. Which of the following is NOT a link in the chain of infection?

    d) Decontamination

2. Which of the following are possible signs and symptoms of a wound infection?

    c) Exudate, redness, pain

3. Which of the following micro-organisms is considered to be part of the normal flora of the skin?

    a) *Staphylococcus epidermidis*

4. What is the main route of transmission of MRSA?

    d) Contact

5. Which of the following sites is normally sterile?

    d) The bladder

6. Which of the following is NOT a virulence factor?

    a) A phagocyte

Further reading

Engelkirk, PG and Burton, GRW (2007) *Burton's Microbiology for the Health Sciences*, 8th edition. Baltimore: Lippincott Williams & Wilkins.

This has some interesting sections for students with a particular interest in microbiology who wish to study beyond what is required for the purposes of their pre-registration programme.

Gould, D and Brooker, C (2008) *Infection Prevention and Control: Applied Microbiology for Healthcare*, 2nd edition. Basingstoke: Palgrave Macmillan.

This is a good companion for this text and is an easy to read textbook.

Peate, I and Nair, M (2011) *Fundamentals of Anatomy and Physiology for Student Nurses*. Oxford: Wiley-Blackwell.

This book is specifically for nursing students and is therefore easier to understand than more complex books.

Watson, R (2011) *Anatomy and Physiology for Nurses*. Oxford: Elsevier Ltd.

This is a suggested anatomy and physiology book written specifically for nurses.

Useful websites

www.microbiologyonline.org.uk

This website provides links to basic information about microbiology which will support your learning.

www.sccm.org/Documents/SSC-Guidelines.pdf

This is a link to the 2012 guidelines on sepsis management which provide in-depth information about the condition and its management.

http://nfsuk.org.uk

This is a link to the Lee Spark NF Foundation website where you can find information about necrotising fasciitis.

Chapter 3
Bacteria

Chapter aims

After reading this chapter, you will be able to:

- Understand bacterial classification.
- Describe some of the important structures which make up a bacterial cell.
- Identify some of the important bacteria in healthcare.
- Describe some of the issues relating to antimicrobial resistance.
- Provide an overview of some of the resistant bacteria in healthcare.

In the previous chapter you were introduced to microbiology, including the chain of infection. One of the links in the chain of infection is the causative micro-organism. In this chapter we will be looking as micro-organisms known as bacteria which can cause infection in people. Initially there will be a brief overview of the structure of bacterial cells. We will then go on to consider different classification systems for bacteria used in healthcare before then looking further at some important bacteria which you might need to know more about in your role as a nurse. The chapter will conclude by considering antibiotic resistance, including some of the more significant antibiotic resistant bacteria in healthcare. Throughout the chapter there are activities and scenarios to enable you to test your knowledge and apply your knowledge of bacteria to nursing practice.

Bacterial cell structure and function

The human body is full of bacteria; there are actually more bacteria cells in the body than there are human cells and there are more bacteria in the intestines than there are people on earth!

When reading microbiology books as a nursing student, bacterial cell structure can become very confusing. This book aims to provide you with adequate information and knowledge to assist in your programme of study both academically and clinically. For students who wish to study in more detail, information is provided about further reading at the end of this chapter. In some books you will also see bacteria referred to as **procaryotes**. This is a term in micro-biology used to refer to the more simple organisms such as bacteria and archaea, the latter being of no significance in healthcare. The other term that you may read is **eucaryotes** which refers to the more complicated micro-organisms such as fungi and protozoa. Viruses and prions are not considered to fall within either of these groups. These are considered in Chapters 4 and 5.

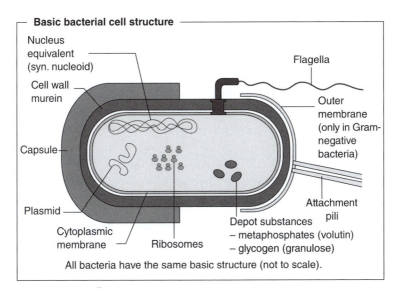

Figure 3.1: Bacterial cell structure

When considering bacterial structure, we need to look at the following:

- The cell membrane – this is generally surrounded by a cell wall and in some bacteria also has an additional outer layer.

- **Cytoplasm** with **ribosomes** and a nuclear region – in some bacteria there are also granules and vesicles.

- External structures which differ between bacteria such as capsules and **flagella**.

If we take these structures in order, we now need to briefly consider the cell wall, cell membrane, cytoplasm, ribosomes, nuclear region, granules, **vesicles** and external structures.

The cell wall

This is semi-rigid and surrounds the cell membrane in most bacteria. It maintains the shape of the cell and prevents the cell from bursting when fluids enter it. The cell wall does not generally play a significant role in preventing the entry of materials into the cell as it is very porous. The cell wall's components include **peptidoglycan** (which forms a supporting net-type structure around the cell that looks like layers of a chain-link fence). There are several different molecules within peptidoglycan, but the main thing to remember is that Gram-positive bacteria have an additional molecule that Gram-negative bacteria do not contain – this is one of the aspects that makes the cell walls different in these two groups of bacteria.

The outer membrane of the cell wall has two layers and is generally found in Gram-negative bacteria (see later in chapter), attached to the peptidoglycan by a layer of **lipoprotein** molecules. This outer membrane also contains **lipopolysaccharide** which can be used to identify Gram-negative bacteria.

The periplasmic space is the gap between the cell membrane and the cell wall and is most commonly observed in Gram-negative bacteria. However, Gram-positive bacteria do have **periplasms** which, in both groups of bacteria, contain digestive enzymes and transport proteins which play a role in destroying substances which may be harmful and transporting metabolites into the bacterial cytoplasm.

The cell membrane

Bacterial cell membranes have the same basic structure as that of other cells within the body. The membrane consists mainly of proteins and **phospholipids**. The main function of the bacterial cell membrane is to control the movement of materials into and out of the cell – some antibiotics actually kill bacteria by causing their cell membranes to leak. Further information about the physical structure of the cell membrane can be found by searching online for the term 'fluid-mosaic model' which is what we currently understand to be the structure of a cell membrane. The best websites to use are reputable ones such as the biology online website (see end of chapter).

Cytoplasm

This is a semi-fluid substance found inside the cell membrane. This is what bacterial cells consist of primarily. It is mainly composed of water with the other components including enzymes, proteins, **lipids** and carbohydrates. Chemical reactions occur within the cytoplasm.

Ribosomes

These are found within the cytoplasm and consist of **RNA** and protein. They are sometimes found in chains within the cytoplasm and are sites for protein **synthesis**.

Nuclear region

While some micro-organisms have an actual nucleus, this is not the case in bacterial cells. Instead they have a nuclear region or **nucleoid** which consists mainly of **DNA** with some RNA and protein. This is found within the cytoplasm of the cell.

Granules and vesicles

Granules are also found within the cytoplasm and they contain substances such as **glycogen** or **polyphosphate** which are used for energy and metabolic purposes. Vesicles are enclosed by a membrane and are also called vacuoles. Some are filled with gas and others store energy.

Endospores

Some bacteria produce a resting stage called an endospore. Examples of bacteria which do this include *Clostridium difficile*, discussed later in this chapter. Endospores are very resistant to heat, drying and some disinfectants which makes them difficult to destroy in the environment.

Flagella

Around half of bacteria are capable of movement, usually by means of an appendage called a flagella. Bacteria can have one, two or multiple flagella. Spirochetes (see later) have **endoflagella** which extend beyond the cell wall.

Pili

These are tiny projections but are not involved in movement. There are two types of pili which are used to attach bacteria to surfaces: conjugation pili which are found in some groups of bacteria provide a pathway for the transfer of DNA which can contribute to antibiotic resistance; and attachment pili which help bacteria to attach to cell surfaces, enhancing colonisation and contributing to the **pathogenicity** of some bacteria.

Capsule

This is a protective structure secreted by certain bacteria – the chemical structure is dependent on the bacterium which forms it. When bacteria with capsules invade a person the capsule prevents some of the immune response from destroying the bacteria.

Bacterial classification

Bacteria are generally classified according to their shape, staining and oxygen requirements.

Bacterial shape

- Cocci – these bacteria consist of spherical-shaped cells which may appear in pairs, chains or clusters. Examples of bacteria with this shape are *Staphylococcus aureus*, *Streptococcus pyogenes* and *Neisseria meningitides*.

- Bacilli (including **vibrios**) – these are rod-shaped bacteria – vibrios are small curved rods. Bacteria in this group include *Escherichia coli*, *Campylobacter jejuni* (which causes gastro-enteritis) and *Clostridium difficile*.

- Spirochetes – these are slender helical cells which move by endoflagella. *Treponema pallidum* (which causes syphilis) and leptospira are both spirochetes.

Bacterial staining

Gram staining is a technique used in the laboratory to identify different types of bacteria. Essentially there are four different reactions to Gram staining: bacteria whose cell walls retain a crystal violet stain, known as Gram-positive bacteria; those whose cell wall does not retain the stain and turn pink, known as Gram-negative bacteria; those which do not stain or stain poorly, known as Gram-nonreactive bacteria; and those which stain unevenly which are referred to as Gram-variable bacteria. In healthcare the terms Gram-positive and Gram-negative are the ones which are commonly used and which you will hear the most as a nurse. Most bacteria are therefore generally referred to as either Gram-positive or Gram-negative.

Oxygen requirements

Some bacteria need oxygen to survive, some survive best in environments which are free from oxygen and some can survive in either environment.

Aerobic bacteria are those which require oxygen; anaerobic bacteria are those which do not require oxygen and facultative aerobic bacteria can survive either with or without oxygen.

At this stage you may be wondering why a nurse needs to know what shape bacteria are when viewed under a microscope. After all, you do not look under the microscope in the laboratory and your main interest is in identifying what infection the patient has so that it can be treated and managed appropriately. The shape does not help you in this endeavour. Or does it? Consider the scenario below.

Scenario

Trevor is a 48-year-old man who has recently had a vascular graft which has led to there being a surgical wound in his groin. The nurse notices that the site is looking infected – it is red, painful and there is pus production, plus Trevor is pyrexial at 38.5°C. As a consequence of this, blood tests including blood cultures (see Chapter 6) and a wound swab are obtained. It will take around three days for the results of the swab to be available so that appropriate antibiotic treatment can be prescribed.

> *Later that night, Trevor becomes increasingly unwell, with a pyrexia of 39°C and a tachycardia of 110 bpm. He is experiencing rigors and has clammy skin, looking pale on observation. As yet there is no news from the laboratory about the micro-organisms causing the infection in Trevor's graft site. At this stage, the nurses are concerned about his condition and call the doctor who contacts the on-call microbiologist for advice. At this stage the laboratory has been able to identify that the infection is caused by a spherical bacterium. This enables the doctors to rule out bacteria of any other shape as causing the infection. Treatment options can therefore be focused on antibiotics which treat cocci (spherical shaped) rather than any other shape of organism. The microbiologist therefore advises the team caring for Trevor of the best option for treatment so that this can be prescribed. At a later stage, Gram staining results come through which means that the treatment can be refined further in order to target the cause of Trevor's infection.*

It should be clear from the scenario above that knowing the shape and staining requirements of bacteria can allow targeted treatment for seriously ill patients where the exact organism is not yet known, but the patient cannot wait any longer for appropriate treatment.

Considering these three ways to classify bacteria, if for example we knew that an infection organism was a Gram-negative anaerobic bacillus, we would know that its cell wall stained pink on Gram testing, it does not require oxygen and it is rod-shaped. This would enable the microbiology laboratory to greatly narrow the focus of treatment for an infected patient.

Gram-positive bacteria

Later in the chapter, Table 3.1 gives the general bacteria within each classification in terms of Gram-negative and Gram-positive according to whether they are cocci or rods. Not all of these will be covered in this chapter; instead we will consider those of most importance in healthcare to provide you with an overview of them in preparation for caring for such patients in practice. Knowledge of these bacteria will enable you to explain things better to patients and their relatives and to understand treatment decisions made for your patients in terms of antibiotic therapy. In this section we will therefore be talking in more detail about some of these bacteria.

Staphylococci

All these are cocci and stain purple in the laboratory. Staphylococci are considered to be coagulase positive or negative. This is a type of test in the laboratory which is used to distinguish between one type of staphylococcus and another. In terms of nursing practice, you need to be aware of this so that you understand what laboratory or medical staff are referring to when they say the term 'coag neg staph'. *Staphylococcus epidermidis* and *Staphylococcus saprophyticus* are both coagulase negative whereas *Staphylococcus aureus* is coagulase positive. Generally when healthcare workers talk about 'coag neg staph' they are referring to *Staphylococcus epidermidis*. This is particularly talked about in relation to contamination of blood cultures obtained from patients when staph would not generally require treatment, whereas if the blood culture contained 'coag positive staph' it would be considered to be more significant in terms of treatment requirements.

Staphylococcus aureus

This is a Gram-positive coccus which occurs in clusters when seen under the microscope. It is thought that around 30% of the population is colonised with this bacterium somewhere on their body. It can therefore be a significant endogenous source of infection in relation to surgical and other wounds. Its main route of transmission is direct contact and therefore the precautions detailed in Chapter 8 are required as with all patients. *Staphylococcus aureus* can cause various infections including wound infections in surgical sites, boils etc. Some isolates of *Staphylococcus aureus* produce toxins. For example, around half produce enterotoxins which can contaminate food and cause food poisoning. It can also produce toxic shock syndrome toxin (TSST-1) which causes toxic shock syndrome. This is a life-threatening condition which causes toxins to damage the tissues and disturb the function of body organs.

Other infections which can be caused by *Staphylococcus aureus* include acute **endocarditis** (usually but not always associated with intravenous drug use), **septicaemia**, pneumonia and scalded skin syndrome (resulting from toxin production). This bacterium therefore causes disease by entering tissues and causing damage or by the production of toxins.

Depending on laboratory reports, *Staphylococcus aureus* may be treated with a variety of antibiotics including those in the penicillin group. However, there is widespread resistance in the UK and this can result in this bacterium becoming meticillin (now flucloxacillin) resistant which means that is becomes an MRSA (meticillin resistant *Staphylococcus aureus*) (see later in this chapter). You may also see the term 'MSSA' written – this is meticillin sensitive *Staphylococcus aureus* and is therefore standard *Staphylococcus aureus* which is sensitive to flucloxacillin.

Staphylococcus epidermidis

This is a Gram-positive coccus which is significant in healthcare primarily as it causes infections in medical devices such as prosthetic joints, catheters, heart valves and so on. It is also considered to be a common skin contaminant in **blood cultures** if they are not obtained correctly. It is primarily considered to be part of the normal flora of the skin in the majority of people, hence its potential for contamination of other body systems. It produces a material sometimes referred to as 'slime' which assists in its adherence to prosthetic surfaces such as intravenous catheters – it therefore acts as a barrier to agents such as **antiseptics**. It does have a low virulence but also demonstrates resistance to some antibiotics.

Staphylococcus saprophyticus

This is primarily significant in the urinary tract as it is the second most common cause of urinary tract infections – it particularly affects young females who are sexually active, probably as a result of its occurrence in the vagina as normal flora. It is sensitive to most antibiotics and is therefore relatively easy to treat.

Streptococci

There are various bacteria in this group including *Streptococcus agalactiae*, *Streptococcus bovis*, *Streptococcus mutans*, *Streptococcus pneumonia* and *Streptococcus pyogenes*. These bacteria are generally classified by their haemolytic properties (so may be referred to as alpha-haemolytic or beta-haemolytic for example); or by what is called the Lancefield groupings (groups A to U, with A and B being most significant in healthcare as they are the most commonly encountered).

The most important to consider in healthcare are group A beta-haemolytic streptococci (*Streptococcus pyogenes*); group B beta-haemolytic streptococci (*Streptococcus agalactiae*) and alpha-haemolytic streptococci (*Streptococcus pneumonia*) as these cause the most infections (PHE, 2015).

Streptococcus pyogenes is one of the most frequently seen bacterial pathogens which affects humans worldwide. This bacterium does not survive well in the environment and uses skin and mucous membranes as a reservoir. Respiratory droplets can also spread infection from one person to another. It is a major cause of cellulitis and can also cause pharyngitis, tonsillitis, impetigo (a skin condition), erysipelas (another skin condition which causes redness and swelling), puerperal sepsis after pregnancy, invasive disease such as necrotising fasciitis, rheumatic fever, toxic shock syndrome and glomerulonephritis. The most common treatment is penicillin as it has not yet developed resistance to this antibiotic.

Streptococcus agalactiae can be found in the male and female genital tract of carriers as well as in the gastro-intestinal tract. It is often also referred to as group B streptococcus. Transmission can occur from affected women to their baby during delivery. It is a leading cause of meningitis and septi-caemia in neonates. Most can be treated with penicillin or ampicillin. Some NHS organisations screen pregnant women for *Streptococcus agalactiae* so that treatment can be given during labour or prior to this to minimise the risk of spread to the infant. However, this is not recommended by the Royal College of Obstetricians and Gynaecologists in the UK.

Streptococcus pneumoniae causes most disease among young children, the elderly, smokers and those with certain chronic conditions. It can be found in the nasopharynx of many otherwise healthy people. It can cause infections such as pneumonia, otitis media, sepsis and meningitis (the latter having a high mortality rate). There is a high level of resistance to penicillin in this bacterium, but it can generally be treated by a group of antibiotics called cephalosporins. There is a pneumo-coccal vaccine available and it is part of the childhood immunisation programme in the UK.

Enterococci

The main enterococci to consider are *Enterococcus faecium* and *Enterococcus faecalis*. Enterococci used to be considered to be group D streptococci, but are now seen to be separate. Enterococci are part of the normal flora, but can also colonise areas such as the skin and mucous membranes in the mouth. They can be a cause of healthcare-associated infection, usually in situations where the person has lowered resistance or when there is interference with the function of the gastro-intestinal or genito-urinary tract (such as catheter insertion). Enterococci can cause urinary tract infections, sepsis, endocarditis, abscesses in the abdomen and infections of the biliary tract. Many enterococci are resistant to multiple antibiotics and therefore laboratory sensitivity tests are important in patients with this infection.

Clostridia

This group includes *Clostridium botulinum* (which causes botulism), *Clostridium difficile* (see below), *Clostridium perfringens* (which can cause cellulitis, gas gangrene and food poisoning) and *Clostridium tetani* (which causes tetanus).

Of particular significance in healthcare is *Clostridium difficile* which is the most common cause of antibiotic-associated diarrhoea. *Clostridium difficile* is a spore forming bacterium and can therefore survive on environmental surfaces for a significant period of time. When such patients are symptomatic, it is usually the policy to isolate them in a single room to minimise the risk of cross-infection. The infection can be treated with metronidazole or vancomycin depending on severity but longer courses than is usually recommended are required (usually at least 10 days). In addition, other treatments including probiotics, rifampicin, fusidic acid and rifaximin may be used (PHE, 2013c; HPS, 2014). Public Health England produced updated guidance on the management and treatment of this infection in 2013. It is worth looking at this document (see further reading at the end of this chapter) to compare what you see in practice with what the document advises. There is currently some disagreement in the literature about whether alcohol hand rub (see Chapter 8) can be used for hand hygiene when caring for patients with *Clostridium difficile* – the current recommendation in epic3 (Loveday et al., 2014) is to use soap and water rather than alcohol hand rub in patients with a gastro-intestinal illness, and this would include *Clostridium difficile*.

Gram-negative bacteria

Again it would be useful to refer to Table 3.1 where you can see identified several Gram-negative bacteria. This section will be considering some of these in more detail.

Escherichia coli

E. coli is the commonest cause of urinary tract infections in the UK. It is a Gram-negative rod and can cause gastro-intestinal infections, often from food poisoning. This bacterium can cause mild to severe infection, sometimes resulting in death. It can be associated with haemalytic uraemic syndrome (HUS) which has a severe effect on the kidneys and causes serious illness.

Neisseria (including *Neisseria meningitidis* and *Neisseria gonorrhoea*)

This group of bacteria can cause a range of infections. The main ones to consider are *Neisseria meningitidis* which causes meningococcal disease including meningitis and *Neisseria gonorrhoea* which causes a sexually transmitted infection. Both of these are treated with antibiotics.

Klebsiella

These are large bacilli. *Klebsiella penumoniae* and *Klebsiella oxytoca* both cause necrotising pneumonia in individuals who may be compromised by issues such as alcoholism, diabetes or chronic lung conditions. *Klebsiella pneumoniae* also causes urinary tract infections and bacteraemia. *Klebsiella* species have developed levels of resistance to antibiotics referred to later in this chapter.

Acinetobacter

At this stage what you need to know about *Acinetobacter* is that they are an important issue in relation to healthcare-associated infection, in particular in areas such as the intensive therapy unit/intensive care unit where the bacteria can contaminate the environment including environmental surfaces.

Mycobacterium tuberculosis

This is the bacterium responsible for tuberculosis (TB). This is commonly considered to be an infection of the lungs, but TB can affect other parts of the body including lymph nodes, the kidneys and bones. Patients with pulmonary TB are usually isolated until they have been receiving continuous treatment for two weeks or, if at home, advised to stay at home and make no new contacts until they have received their initial two weeks of treatment. Staff and visitors do not generally need to wear masks for routine activities, but masks are recommended for staff during cough producing procedures. Where the TB is multi-drug resistant (or MDR-TB), additional precautions such as use of masks for all patient contact and stricter isolation may be advocated in some NHS Trusts, depending on local policy (see Chapters 8 and 9).

Other groups of bacteria

Mycoplasma

These include *Mycoplasma hominis, Mycoplasma incognitus, Mycoplasma pneumoniae* and *Mycoplasma urealyticum.* The most important of these is *Mycoplasma pneumoniae.* It is transmitted by respiratory droplets and causes a lower respiratory tract infection, generally an atypical pneumonia. It can also cause bronchitis, pharyngitis and otitis media. Treatment can be with antibiotics such as doxycycline but the micro-organism can persist in the respiratory tract for long periods after symptomatic recovery.

Spirochetes

This group causes infections such as *Borrelia burgdorferi* (which causes Lyme disease and is treated by amoxicillin or doxycycline), *Leptospira interrogans* (which causes leptospirosis and is treated with penicillin in the early stages of the disease) and *Treponema pallidum* (which causes syphilis and is treated with penicillin).

Obligate intracellular parasites

This term can be confusing due to the word 'parasite' when this is a different classification of micro-organism – however, parasitic bacteria are still bacteria rather than parasites. They include *Chlamydia* (*Chlamydia pneumoniae* which causes pharyngitis, bronchitis and pneumonia, *Chlamydia psittaci* which usually infects the lower respiratory tract and *Chlamydia trachomatis* which causes genito-urinary and eye infections), *Coxiella, Ehrlichia* and *Rickettsia.* Chlamydiae are sensitive to a number of broad-spectrum antibiotics.

Gram-positive cocci	Gram-positive rods	Gram-negative cocci	Gram-negative rods (inc. vibrios)
Staphylococci (clusters) Streptococci (chains or pairs) Peptostreptococci Enterococci	Corynebacteria *Bacillus* *Listeria* *Propionibacterium* *Lactobacillus* *Erysipelothrix* *Clostridia* (spore-forming)	*Neisseria* (pairs) *Moraxella* *Acinetobacter*	*Campylobacter* *Enterobacter* *Escherichia* *Helicobacter* *Klebsiella* *Bartonella* *Bordetella* *Brucella* *Francisella* *Haemophilus* *Legionella* *Pasteurella* *Pseudomonas aeruginosa* *Yersinia pestis* *Bacteroides* Mycobacteria (Gram-variable) *Proteus* *Salmonella*
	Mycoplasma	**Spirochetes (Gram-negative)**	**Obligate intracellular parasites**
	Hominis Incognitus Pneumonia Ureaplasma	*Treponema pallidum* *Borrelia* *Leptospira*	*Coxiella* *Ehrlichia* *Rickettsia* *Chlamydia*

Table 3.1: Classification of bacteria according to shape and Gram staining

Now that you have considered this table, it is time to quickly review what you have learned so far!

Activity 3.1 — *Critical thinking*

Consider the following scenario. This will be relevant to all fields of nursing as all fields may undertake placement in the A&E department.

James presents himself at the accident and emergency department complaining of a swollen, red and painful left leg which he states is now leaking green fluid. He has a pyrexia of 38.5° and a tachycardia of 106 bpm. A swab is obtained and sent to the laboratory to identify what micro-organism might be causing the signs and symptoms of infection. Later

James's condition deteriorates in the department and his blood pressure drops. The senior staff are suspecting sepsis (which you have covered in the previous chapter). It is therefore important at this stage to focus the antibiotic therapy as closely as possible. The doctor rings the microbiology laboratory to try to gain further information and is told that the pus from the wound demonstrates bacteria which are Gram-positive cocci. Considering what you have learned so far, and considering which Gram-positive cocci might cause skin or wound infections, what are the possible bacteria which might be causing James's infection?

Answers can be found at the end of this chapter.

Antibiotics and antimicrobial resistance

Antibiotics and **antimicrobials** are not the same thing, though sometimes you may hear the terms used interchangeably. Antimicrobials inhibit or destroy pathogens such as bacteria, viruses, fungi or parasites. They do this by one of several means including the inhibition of cell wall synthesis; damage to cell membranes; inhibition of synthesis of nucleic acid; inhibition of protein synthesis; or inhibition of enzyme activity. Some antimicrobial agents are antibiotics which are considered to be either bacteriostatic, meaning they inhibit the growth of bacteria; or bactericidal which means they kill bacteria. You will hear antibiotics referred to as narrow-spectrum or broad-spectrum. Narrow-spectrum antibiotics may only act on Gram-positives or Gram-negatives but not both – those which act on both are considered to be broad-spectrum. Table 3.2 provides some examples of antibiotics that you may see in practice and how they work. More information about different antibiotics and how they work can be found in pharmacology text books, some of which are detailed in the further reading section at the end of this chapter.

Many factors contribute towards antibiotic resistance. These include prescribing doses that are lower than required, poor compliance of patients with antibiotic treatment such as not completing the course, inappropriate use of antibiotics when they are not needed, incorrect choice of antibiotic (such as prescribing an antibiotic that is not appropriate for treating the presenting infection) or indiscriminate use of antibiotics without a prescription, which occurs in many countries.

Activity 3.2   *Critical thinking*

Consider the reasons why patients do not comply fully with taking their prescribed course of antibiotics. What reasons can you think of?

What do you think nurses can do in practice to prevent antibiotic resistance?

Possible answers can be found at the end of this chapter.

As you will have recognised from this activity, there are many reasons why patients do not always comply with antibiotic courses. However, poor compliance can contribute towards antibiotic resistance which nurses need to help to address.

Antibiotic	How it acts
Cephalosporins Imipenum Penicillins, e.g. amoxicillin, ampicillin, piperacillin Vancomycin	Inhibits cell wall synthesis
Chloramphenicol Clindamycin Erythromycin Tetracycline	Inhibits protein synthesis
Rifampicin Quinolones and fluoroquinolones, e.g. ciprofloxacin	Inhibits nucleic acid synthesis
Colistin	Disrupts cell membranes
Sulfonamides Trimethoprim	Inhibits enzyme activity

Table 3.2: Some antibiotics and their actions

As a nurse, there are many actions that may be taken to minimise antimicrobial resistance.

Activity 3.3   *Critical thinking*

Go to the Royal College of Nursing website and access their 2014 publication 'Antimicrobial Resistance' (RCN, 2014a). Consider what it says about the contribution of nursing to the prevention of antimicrobial resistance.

Suggested answers can be found at the end of this chapter.

As can be seen from this document, nursing and nurses have a valuable contribution to make in the fight against resistance. However, while we need to focus on prevention, we also need to acknowledge that as nurses we care for patients with drug resistant infections. We will now consider some of these in the healthcare setting.

Antibiotic resistant bacteria in healthcare

MRSA (Gram-positive cocci, coagulase positive)

MRSA is a *Staphylococcus aureus* which is resistant to the antibiotic meticillin. We no longer use this antibiotic in the UK and instead we consider MRSA as demonstrating resistance to the antibiotic flucloxacillin. MRSA will also be resistant to all penicillins and all cephalosporins (a group of antibiotics) due to their repeated use in the population. MRSA causes the same infections as

Staphylococcus aureus does, but the treatment options are more limited. In the UK it is mandatory for NHS organisations to report all their cases of MRSA bacteraemia (bloodstream infections). There has been a lot of emphasis in recent years on reducing cases of MRSA bloodstream infections and the target for reduction was reached. However, MRSA continues to be a problem in many healthcare settings, causing surgical site and wound infections, chest infections, urinary tract infections and colonisation of body sites such as the nose, axillae and groin area. In many situations, patients are screened for MRSA on admission to hospital, usually involving a nose swab. While different hospitals may have different groups of patients that they screen for MRSA based on local need, the Department of Health (2014) currently recommends that screening on admission is performed on patients who have previously been identified to be MRSA positive and patients admitted to high-risk units (including vascular, renal, neuro- and cardiothoracic surgery, bone marrow transplant units, orthopaedics and all intensive care units). Patients who are MRSA positive may be colonised, infected or both. Colonisation may be treated to prevent it causing infection in the colonised person or to prevent its spread to other patients. The Department of Health recommends that all patients admitted to hospital who are identified as being colonised with MRSA should be treated. This is undertaken in a variety of ways using decolonisation or suppression treatment which includes topical antiseptic washes and shampoo, powders and nasal ointments. Suppression regimes aim to reduce MRSA below the detection level at the time of risk, to decrease chance of infection and spread, such as prior to surgical procedures. Infection with MRSA is treated depending on the antibiotics that the particular strain is sensitive to.

Case study

Fred is a 68-year-old man being cared for at home by his wife. He receives regular visits from the district nurse to dress an ulcer on his right lower leg. The ulcer has repeatedly been infected with MRSA which each time is successfully treated with antibiotics. The nurse decides to undertake a full screen for MRSA to see if this is a source of the re-infection. On this screen MRSA is identified as colonising his nose, axillae and groins which the nurse realises is providing an endogenous source for his leg ulcer infections. In order to prevent more recurring infections in his leg ulcer, which are likely being re-infected from the endogenous source of his own colonised body sites, he is given topical decolonisation therapy which the nurse educates him on how to apply. This helps to reduce the MRSA from his nose, axillae and groins and prevents re-infection of his leg ulcer again.

As can be seen from the above scenario, decolonisation treatment can be very important for the welfare of the affected patient. Colonisation with MRSA is not always treated, particularly outside the hospital setting where it does not pose a risk to others, as it may not be beneficial and treatment can cause side effects. However, in the above case it is warranted as though it is not always effective, it can often help to reduce the risk.

When patients have MRSA, usual standard precautions should be applied (see Chapter 8) and some patients may be isolated on a risk assessment basis, though the Department of Health advises that all known or suspected cases, such as those previously identified as MRSA positive, should be isolated. In reality, the allocation of single rooms in the NHS can be problematic as there are not always enough to meet demand, so there may be several patients with different infections requiring isolation at the same time. In these cases, single rooms are allocated on a risk assessment basis, often with the advice of the infection prevention and control nurse (see Chapter 7). In terms of caring for patients with MRSA, the infection prevention and control management should be the same as with patients with other infections in terms of standard precautions and isolation based on risk assessment. The difference is in terms of admission screening for MRSA, screening body sites for colonisation once a body site is found to be infected, and the tagging of notes and electronic records in some organisations so that patients previously found to have MRSA can be identified on readmission. In some organisations, patients with MRSA are moved to the end of lists, such as in the operating theatre, for procedures such as surgery but if usual precautions are applied this should not be necessary (Agha, 2012) as the standard precautions discussed in Chapter 8 should minimise the risk of cross-infection.

Activity 3.4   *Evidence-based practice and research*

Look at the MRSA policy in the organisation where you are currently on placement. Look at the following areas:

- Who is screened for MRSA on admission?
- Who is isolated when they have MRSA and why?

There is no answer provided for this activity as the answers will vary between organisations. It may be useful to discuss this activity with a local infection prevention and control nurse.

You may have identified from this activity that there are differences between the local policy and what the Department of Health advises. You might also have noticed that practice in the clinical area differs from that suggested within the policy due to resource restrictions. This is something to consider as a nurse when dealing with infections which require additional precautions such as screening and isolation.

VRE/GRE (Gram-positive cocci)

Glycopeptide-resistant enterococci (GRE) are enterococci that are resistant to glycopeptide antibiotics (vancomycin and teicoplanin). GRE are sometimes also referred to as VRE (vancomycin-resistant enterococci).

The two most common species of GRE are *Enterococcus faecalis* and *Enterococcus faecium*. Infections caused by GRE mainly occur in hospital patients, particularly those who are immunocompromised, have had previous treatment with antibiotics such as glycopeptides, are in hospital for long periods and are on specialist units such as a renal or intensive care unit.

Colonisation is much more common than infection with GRE. If a patient is suspected of having GRE a full screen is usually required which can consist of stool samples (or rectal swabs), wound swabs, urine specimen if a catheter is in situ, and a central venous catheter site swab if one is in situ. Usual standard precautions apply as detailed in Chapter 8. It is also recommended that patients with GRE are isolated.

Extended spectrum beta lactamases (Gram-negative rods)

Bacteria that produce enzymes called extended-spectrum beta-lactamases (ESBLs) are resistant to many penicillin and cephalosporin antibiotics and often to other types of antibiotic. The two main bacteria that produce ESBLs are *Escherichia coli* (*E. coli*) and *Klebsiella* species. Most of the infections have occurred in people with other long-term conditions, and in elderly people. Patients who have been taking antibiotics or who have been previously hospitalised are mainly affected. As with other infections, standard precautions apply and it is recommended that patients with these infections are isolated in a single room. *E. coli* and *Klebsiella* are not always considered to be ESBLs – this is only the case when they produce the enzymes.

Carbapenemase producing Enterobacteriaceae (Gram-negative rods)

Carbapenemase producing Enterobacteriaceae (also sometimes referred to as carbapenamase producing **coliforms**) are Gram-negative rods which are increasingly becoming a problem in healthcare. Enterobacteriaceae include organisms such as *Klebsiella*, *E. coli*, *Acinetobacter* and *Pseudomonas aureginosa* – when these organisms produce an enzyme called carbapenemase which results in levels of resistance to a group of antibiotics known as carbapenems, this means they are referred to as CPE. You may hear various acronyms in practice such as CRE, KPV, NDM, VIM and so on – these are all organisms within the CPE group, but the use of different terms can be confusing. As you can see, some of these organisms are referred to in different ways depending on what enzymes they produce and therefore *E. coli* could just be 'e. coli', could be an ESBL or could be a CPE. Obviously this can be quite confusing, but the main message to remember is that standard precautions and isolation are generally required. Public Health England produced a tool kit in 2013 to provide NHS organisations with guidance on how to manage patients with CPE (PHE, 2013d). This includes a decision tree about which patients to screen for CPE via a rectal swab and what action to take if the patient is positive. It is generally recommended that patients with CPE are isolated. The usual standard precautions are applied. Treatment options are limited as with other antibiotic resistant organisms but treatment is both available and effective in the UK.

Activity 3.5   *Evidence-based practice and research*

Go to the following website:

www.gov.uk/government/publications/carbapenemase-producing-enterobacteriaceae-early-detection-management-and-control-toolkit-for-acute-trust

(Continued)

continued . . . •

Access the resources available about CPE from Public Health England and consider how you might use these in practice.

There is no answer provided for this activity as the use of the toolkit will depend on the type of organisation and ward that you are currently working on. It might also be useful for you to look at local policies and procedures relating to CPE management to identify what they do. Again, you could also speak to a member of the infection prevention and control team.

As can be seen from the above activity, PHE has determined that CPE is a priority and has provided a lot of information for healthcare workers about how to manage it, from ground level upwards.

Throughout this chapter we have considered bacteria, antimicrobial resistance and bacteria of specific importance in healthcare settings. It is now time to review what you have learned by working through the following activity.

Activity 3.6   *Multiple choice questions*

1. Which of the following is a Gram-negative rod?

    a) *Neisseria meningitidis*
    b) Enterococci
    c) *Campylobacter jejuni*
    d) *Clostridium difficile*
    e) *Acinetobacter*

2. Which of the following is a spirochete?

    a) *Staphylococcus aureus*
    b) *Treponema pallidum*
    c) *Escherichia coli*
    d) *Listeria*
    e) *Bordetella pertussis*

3. Name the two most common causes of urinary tract infections:

    a) *Neisseria gonorrhoea* and *Escherichia coli*
    b) *Neisseria gonorrhoea* and *Chlamydia trachomatis*
    c) *Chlamydia trachomatis* and *Escherichia coli*
    d) *Staphylococcus saprophyticus* and *Escherichia coli*
    e) *Staphylococcus saprophyticus* and *Neisseria gonorrhoea*

4. Which of the following antibiotics act on bacterial cell walls?

   a) Penicillin
   b) Rifampicin
   c) Clindamycin
   d) Tetracycline
   e) Chloramphenicol

5. Which bacterial pathogen is the main cause of antibiotic-associated diarrhoea?

   a) MRSA
   b) *Salmonella enteritidis*
   c) *Escherichia coli*
   d) *Clostridium difficile*
   e) *Enterococcus faecalis*

6. Which of the following statements is correct?

   a) *Pseudomonas aureginosa* and *Escherichia coli* are both spherical cells.
   b) *Escherichia coli* is a Gram-negative rod-shaped organism.
   c) *Staphylococcus aureus* is Gram-positive and forms chains of spherical cells.
   d) *Clostridium difficile* is a Gram-negative rod-shaped organism.
   e) *Neisseria gonorrhoea* is a Gram-positive rod-shaped organism.

7. Which enteric organism is associated with haemolytic uraemic syndrome (HUS)?

   a) *Bacillus cereus*
   b) *Clostridium difficile*
   c) *Salmonela enteritidis*
   d) *Escherichia coli*
   e) *Yersinia enterocolitica*

Answers can be found at the end of the chapter.

Chapter summary

Within this chapter you have been introduced to bacteria, considering how they are structured and categorised. We have considered some of the clinically significant bacterial infections that you may come across in the healthcare setting, including some of those which are considered to be antibiotic resistant. We have also briefly looked at antibiotics. The information in this chapter should enable you to speak more knowledgeably with patients and their relatives about their bacterial infections and should act as a basis for infection prevention and control precautions which you apply to your patients and which are covered in Chapters 8 and 9.

Activities: Brief outline answers

Activity 3.1: Critical thinking (pages 46–7)

The bacteria which you should have identified from the table are Staphylococci (clusters), Streptococci (chains or pairs), Peptostreptococci and Enterococci. At this stage you would then consider which of these groups of bacteria would be most likely to cause a wound infection – *Staphylococcus aureus*, for example – and the doctor would prescribe accordingly.

Activity 3.2: Critical thinking (page 47)

- Consider the reasons why patients do not comply fully with taking their prescribed course of antibiotics. What reasons can you think of?
- What do you think nurses can do in practice to prevent antibiotic resistance?

Possible reasons for poor compliance with antibiotic therapy might include **polypharmacy**, lack of motivation to follow treatment regime, a lack of understanding, forgetting to take some of the tablets, boredom if there is prolonged treatment, alcohol or drug dependency, poor taste to medication, size of tablets, antibiotic side effects, cost of prescription, religious or cultural beliefs. Possible actions for nurses that you might have considered could include application of best evidence guidelines, collaboration with other professionals such as doctors and pharmacists, provision of education to patients, questioning the need for antibiotics when they are being prescribed, ensuring that patients do not take antibiotics for less or more time than required, ensure that knowledge of antibiotic resistance is kept up to date and administering antibiotics as prescribed.

Activity 3.3: Critical thinking (page 48)

Possible issues that you might have highlighted related to the RCN Antimicrobial Resistance document should include those around the four key themes which were identified as reducing the demand for antimicrobial treatment (this might include through patient education), enhancing the effectiveness of prescribed antimicrobials (by, for example, ensuring that courses are completed), the provision of specialist infection prevention advice (to patients, carers and more junior staff) and international collaboration and action.

Activity 3.6: MCQs (pages 52–3)

1. Which of the following is a Gram-negative rod?

    c) *Campylobacter jejuni*

2. Which of the following is a spirochete?

    b) *Treponema pallidum*

3. Name the two most common causes of urinary tract infections

    d) *Staphylococcus saprophyticus* and *Escherichia coli*

4. Which of the following antibiotics act on bacterial cell walls?

    a) Penicillin

5. Which bacterial pathogen is the main cause of antibiotic-associated diarrhoea?

    d) *Clostridium difficile*

6. Which of the following statements is correct?

    b) *Escherichia coli* is a Gram-negative, rod-shaped organism

7. Which enteric organism is associated with haemolytic uraemic syndrome (HUS)?

    d) *Escherichia coli*

Further reading

Ashelford, S et al. (2016) *Pathophysiology and Pharmacology for Nursing Students.* London: Sage.

Coia, JE et al. (2006) Guidelines for the control and prevention of methicillin resistant *Staphylococcus aureus* (MRSA) in healthcare facilities. *Journal of Hospital Infection* 63S; S1–S44.

This document provides guidance for hospitals on the management of MRSA.

Cookson, BD et al. (2006) Guidelines for the control of glycopeptide resistant enterococci in hospitals. *Journal of Hospital Infection* 62: 6–21.

This document provides the latest guidance on the management of GRE/VRE and is referred to by PHE as the guidelines to use in practice.

Department of Health (2014) *Implementation of modified admission MRSA screening guidance for NHS.* London: DH.

This provides advice to the NHS on who should be screened for MRSA on admission to hospital. A pdf version can be downloaded at: www.gov.uk/government/uploads/system/uploads/attachment_data/file/345144/Implementation_of_modified_admission_MRSA_screening_guidance_for_NHS.pdf

Public Health England (2013) *Updated guidance on the management and treatment of Clostridium difficile infection.* London: PHE.

Public Health England (2013) *Acute trust toolkit for the early detection, management and control of carbapenemase-producing Enterobacteriaceae.* London: PHE.

This provides the latest guidance to acute hospitals on how to manage CPE.

Royal College of Nursing (2014) *Antimicrobial resistance.* London: RCN.

This document discusses nursing's contribution to the prevention and management of antimicrobial resistance.

RCOG (2012) *The prevention of early-onset neonatal Group B streptococcal disease.* London: RCOG.

This document provides the current guidelines for NHS organisations regarding the management of mothers with group B streptococcal disease to prevent transmission to their babies.

Steer, JA et al. (2012) Guidelines for prevention and control of group A streptococcal infection in acute healthcare and maternity settings in the UK. *Journal of Hospital Infection* 64; 1–18.

This document provides guidance for staff working in hospitals about group A streptococcal management.

Useful websites

www.gov.uk/government/uploads/system/uploads/attachment_data/file/321891/Clostridium_difficile_management_and_treatment.pdf

This provides a link to the PHE guidelines on the treatment and management of *Clostridium difficile.*

www.biology-online.org

This website provides useful information on the fluid-mosaic model of cell membrane structure.

Chapter 4
Viruses

Chapter aims

After reading this chapter, you will be able to:

*   Understand the classification of viruses.
*   Describe some of the common viruses which have an impact on healthcare.
*   Identify some of the treatment options available in the UK.

In the previous chapter we looked at bacteria. Another group of micro-organisms which causes infection in humans is viruses. In this chapter we take a more detailed look at these, including some of the important viruses in healthcare.

Firstly, the chapter considers the classification system used for viruses and the different effects that a virus may have on a person. It then goes on to consider some of the important viruses that you may come across in nursing. It ends by considering treatment options for viruses. Throughout the chapter are case studies and activities to enable you to relate theory to practice and test the knowledge gained throughout the chapter.

There are a million virus particles per millilitre of seawater – for a global total of 10^{30} complete virus particles! Lined up end to end, they would stretch 200 million light years into space. (Suttle, 2007; Breitbart, 2012)

Case study

Jonathan is a six-year-old boy who has a cough, sore throat, runny nose and is coughing up green sputum. His mum is worried as these symptoms have been going on for over a week. She takes Jonathan to see the practice nurse, Janice, at the local health centre and demands antibiotics as she feels that he has suffered enough and wants his symptoms to be treated so that he can feel better. As a qualified nurse, Janice is aware that the symptoms are most likely caused by a cold which is due to a virus. Antibiotics are used for the treatment of bacterial infections and are not effective against viruses. As the majority of viral infections do not require or need treatment, Janice knows that she needs to explain this to Jonathan's mother so that she is happy to take him home without him receiving medicine which will be ineffective.

As a nurse you need to be aware of the differences between viruses and bacteria and how they are managed so that you can advise patients and their relatives accordingly. The information in this chapter will assist you in doing this.

Classification of viruses in healthcare

If you look at various microbiology and virology books, the classification of viruses may be considered differently in each of them. In particular in medical microbiology books aimed at those studying a programme in microbiology, there may be multiple sub-divisions which can be confusing. Viruses are basically grouped into four main categories based on:

1. Their type of nucleic acid (RiboNucleic Acid or DeoxyriboNucleic Acid).

2. Their replication method.

3. The symmetry of their **capsid** (**helical** or **icosahedral**).

4. Whether they are enveloped or not.

In this chapter we will look at classification more simply in terms of two aspects: whether their cells have an envelope surrounding them or not; and whether their nucleic acid contains RNA or DNA. Therefore we finish with four groups: RNA viruses with envelopes, RNA viruses without envelopes, DNA viruses with envelopes and DNA viruses without envelopes. Viruses within each of these groups are shown in Table 4.1. To assist further in understanding the differences between viruses, this table also identifies which are helical and which are icosahedral. As with aspects of bacterial structure discussed in the previous chapter, this is another way of identifying viruses in the laboratory.

DNA enveloped viruses (icosahedral)	DNA non-enveloped viruses (icosahedral)	RNA enveloped viruses (both helical and icosahedral)	RNA non-enveloped viruses (icosahedral)
HERPESVIRIDAE *e.g. herpes simplex, varicella-zoster, cytomegalovirus, Epstein–Barr virus* POXVIRIDAE *e.g. smallpox, molluscum contagiosum* HEPADNAVIRIDAE *e.g. hepatitis B and D*	PARVOVIRIDAE *e.g. parvovirus B19* PAPOVAVIRIDAE *e.g. Human papillomavirus* ADENOVIRIDAE *e.g. conjunctivitis, diarrhoeal illnesses*	FLAVIVIRIDAE (icosahedral) *e.g. dengue fever, yellow fever, hepatitis C* TOGAVIRIDAE (icosahedral) *e.g. rubella* CORONAVIRIDAE (helical) *e.g. SARS* RETROVIRIDAE (icosahedral) *e.g. HIV, HTLV* RABDOVIRIDAE (helical) *e.g. rabies* PARAMYXOVIRIDAE (helical) *e.g. measles, mumps, RSV* ORTHOMYXOVIRIDAE (helical) *e.g. influenza* FILOVIRIDAE (helical) *e.g. Ebola, Marburg* BUNYAVIRIDAE (helical) *e.g. Hantavirus* ARENAVIRIDAE (helical) *e.g. lassa fever*	PICORNAVIRIDAE *e.g. polio, hepatitis A, coxsackie, rhinoviruses, enteroviruses* CALCIVIRIDAE *e.g. norovirus, hepatitis E* REOVIRIDAE *e.g. rotavirus*

Table 4.1: Classification of viruses

The viral envelope

Non-enveloped viruses comprise simply the nucleic acid and a capsid. In enveloped viruses, the capsid is surrounded by an envelope whose membrane contains proteins and lipids. This envelope helps the virus to bind to cells that it wants to infect.

The nucleic acid

The nucleic acid within viral cells may be DNA or RNA. In addition to this it may be single or double stranded. Single stranded RNA viruses are also further divided into those with a positive **polarity** and those with a negative polarity. Nucleic acid contains all the coding needed to make a new virus so it therefore contains all the genetic information to infect a cell. Viral nucleic acid is surrounded by the capsid which protects the genetic material from damage. A complete virus particle with a capsid and nucleic acid, with or without an envelope, is referred to as a virion.

Viral replication

The amount of time that different viruses take to replicate and the number of **progeny virus** they yield differs, but all go through a similar process with two basic stages: the eclipse period and the exponential growth period.

The eclipse period follows the initial attachment of the virus to the host cell. During this period the virus can no longer infect other cells. The period can last between one and twenty hours and during this time there is active synthesis of virus components. Prior to the eclipse period, there is the initial entry and disassembly of the virus and at the end of the period, assembly of the first progeny virion.

During the *exponential growth period,* the number of progeny virus that is produced increases exponentially then reaches a plateau. This stage can take from eight to 72 hours and can yield between 100 and 10,000 virions per infected cell.

There are considered to be several steps in the replication cycles of viruses.

1. Adsorption

When a virus particle initially attaches itself to a host cell, there is an interaction between specific structures on the virion surface and receptors in the host cell membrane which recognise the viral structures.

2. Penetration

This is where the virion passes across the host cell membrane into the cytoplasm.

3. Synthesis

This refers to the process where the virion disassembles, thereby enabling the expression of the viral genes which undertake replication. There is the synthesis of new viral components within the host cell using the metabolic machinery of that cell.

4. Maturation

This step differs depending on whether the infecting agent is a DNA virus or an RNA virus. For both types, however, the information contained in the viral genome is expressed by the use of the cellular make-up of the host cell being infected. Newly synthesised viral components are assembled into complete virions.

5. Assembly and release of progeny viruses

This takes place in the cytoplasm for most RNA viruses and the nucleus for most DNA viruses. Progeny viruses (new virions) are released in different ways from the host cell to infect other cells depending on whether the virus is enveloped or non-enveloped. This stage usually, though not always, results in the death by **lysis** of the host cell (see below).

The effects of viral infection in the infected

There are generally considered to be four responses to infection by a virus:

1. Infections where no progeny virus is produced – this is known as an abortive infection. It has three common causes. Firstly, a normal virus might infect a cell but be lacking in the required compounds, such as enzymes, which are needed for complete replication. Secondly, the virus may have genetically lost the ability to replicate in the type of cell that it infects so the infecting virus is defective. Thirdly, the host cell may die before complete replication of the viral cell.

2. Infections where progeny viruses are released but the host cell is altered rather than killed – this is termed a persistent infection. Viral replication and release does not kill the host cell or interfere with its ability to carry out its function.

3. Infections that result in a latent state in the host cell – in this case there is persistence of the virus genetic material but no production of progeny virus. These viruses can be reactivated at a later date resulting in an actual infection. Sometimes the virus genetic material is integrated into the host cell which can cause alterations in the cell and its growth. This may lead to tumours.

4. Infections where the host cell dies and progeny virus is produced which is most often what occurs – this is known as a lytic infection and results in the shutoff of much of the host cell's syntheses, resulting in cell death.

Viral replication can be a difficult concept to understand. It is therefore useful to look at other ways of learning about it, such as video clips.

Activity 4.1   *Evidence-based practice and research*

Go to **www.youtube.com/watch?v=EqK1CYYQIug** and watch the YouTube video on viral replication – it should take just over ten minutes to watch. Make notes as you go along and identify aspects that you do not understand. Use a virology book (ideas can be found in further reading at the end of this chapter) to find out the information to enable you to more fully understand the process. If you cannot access this clip directly, go to the YouTube home site and enter 'viral replication' as a search term to access several video clips.

There is no answer for this activity.

Hopefully the activity has enabled you to more fully understand how viruses replicate. Now we shall consider different viruses that you may come into contact with in healthcare.

NICE provides a range of resources for some of the viruses to be discussed – these appear on their site as clinical knowledge summaries (CKS) (see website at the end of this chapter) and where one is available, this will be indicated in the discussion in this text. This will enable you as a student nurse to access up-to-date and evidence-based information about the clinical care of patients with specific viral infections.

Enveloped DNA viruses

Viruses within this group are shown in Table 4.1. Within this chapter we will consider some of these so that you can gain a deeper knowledge and understanding of some common, medically important viruses.

Herpesviridae

There are eight known human herpes virus species. All are able to enter a latent phase after initial host infection and be reactivated at a later date.

Herpes simplex virus 1 and 2

Both of these are transmitted by contact with secretions or lesions which contain the virus. HSV-2 primarily causes infections in the genital tract and HSV-1 on the face and oropharyngeal area, with some also occurring in the eyes. Infection with both viruses causes lesions, tiredness and pyrexia. HSV-1 infections can spread to the central nervous system, causing encephalitis which can be life-threatening. HSV-2 infections can be asymptomatic. Both types of infection can reoccur in terms of symptoms with several factors contributing to reactivation including pyrexia and hormone changes. Pain and tingling sensations often occur prior to lesions in reactivation. In HSV-1 reactivations can occur several times per year in some patients, causing 'cold sores' which generally heal within ten days. When HSV-2 is reactivated this can again be asymptomatic and can therefore result in cross-infection to sexual partners or newborn babies. None of the drugs used for HSV can treat latent infection – instead they treat current symptoms and can minimise shedding of the virus in asymptomatic infections to minimise the risk of transmission to others. NICE has a CKS for oral, ocular and genital herpes.

Varicella zoster virus (VZV)

VZV is usually transmitted by respiratory droplets so that the respiratory system is first infected followed by spread via the bloodstream to the lymph nodes. The vesicle-type rash of chicken pox generally occurs between two to three weeks after exposure but those infected can be contagious for a few days before the vesicles appear. The primary infection, known as varicella, is what causes chicken pox. Recurrent infection known as shingles is referred to as herpes zoster. Varicella is much more severe in adults and those who are immuno-compromised. Complications can include pneumonia, encephalitis and hepatic failure. The infection can also be passed from mother to baby in the uterus or, more commonly, during delivery, resulting in developmental abnormalities or a rash. Around 15% of those who have chicken pox find that their infection reactivates at a later date as shingles. The shingles rash is distributed in clusters on skin around branches from a single spinal nerve. Varicella is more commonly treated in neonates and the immuno-compromised but anti-viral agents have limited effectiveness in herpes zoster other than in reducing the time of infection and lessening some of the acute pain experienced. In the hospital setting, patients should be isolated until the vesicles of the rash have crusted over. There are, however, different transmission based precautions applied for chicken pox and shingles as chicken pox is much more transmissible by the airborne route. Such precautions are discussed in Chapters 8 and 9. NICE has a CKS for chicken pox.

Cytomegalovirus (CMV)

Human CMV is a common cause of intrauterine infections and congenital abnormalities – it is therefore primarily significant in pregnancy and additionally in the immuno-compromised (Shenk and Stinski, 2008). CMV occurs commonly in childhood – worldwide up to 90% of people have antibodies to the virus by adulthood. Infection in childhood usually causes no symptoms, but virus can be shed in most body fluids, including tears, meaning that infection can be transmitted to those who are vulnerable. If a pregnant woman acquires CMV for the first time in pregnancy, it can be transmitted to the foetus which can be severe enough to result in foetal death. CMV is also a common opportunistic infection in people who are HIV positive and can cause conditions such as CMV retinitis which can result in visual impairment. It can be difficult to minimise the spread of CMV as so many people have been exposed to it and most body fluids can demonstrate the virus, but general hygiene such as hand washing particularly after going to the toilet and prior to food preparation can be an effective precaution to take. Most cases do not require treatment as the majority of the exposed are asymptomatic. More serious infection may be treated with antiviral drugs (see later in this chapter).

Epstein–Barr virus (EBV)

This is the virus responsible for glandular fever. It is also associated with malignancies such as Burkitt lymphoma and nasopharyngeal cancer. It is transmitted through intimate contact with saliva, hence known as 'the kissing disease'. Isolation is not needed in the hospital setting and the treatments used with other herpes viruses are not effective with EBV.

Hepadnaviridae

Hepatitis B

This virus is transmitted through blood and body fluids, e.g. unprotected sex, sharing needles and mother to baby transmission. It is present in all the body fluids of an infected person including saliva and breast milk. The majority of people with the virus recover from illness without treatment within a few months. Symptoms of acute illness can include pyrexia, tiredness, nausea, a poor appetite, jaundice and dark urine. A minority, however, go on to develop more severe illness which can be fatal. A small proportion of infected people will become chronic carriers of the virus which can lead to liver cancer. There is an immunisation (injection) against hepatitis B which is offered to healthcare workers in the UK. It is also offered to some other groups in some circumstances. The majority of people with hepatitis B recover without needing any treatment and isolation is not routinely needed in hospital. NICE has a CKS for hepatitis B.

Non-enveloped DNA viruses

Parvoviridae

Parvovirus B19 is the only parvovirus that infects humans. It can result in several diseases. It can cause transient aplastic crisis in patients with sickle cell disease. It can also result in polyarthritis in adults. It can cause foetal death if caught in pregnancy. It is however, most commonly known for causing a childhood condition called erythema infectiosum, also known as fifth disease or slapped cheek syndrome. It is most infectious prior to symptoms beginning and isolation in hospital is therefore of no value. Though it is transmitted by the airborne route, once symptoms have developed and the need for isolation is evident, it is no longer infectious. NICE has a CKS for this virus.

Papovaviridae

Human papillomavirus (HPV)

There are over a hundred species of HPV and all induce lesions. Of particular significance is the species which can progress to malignancy such as that which causes cervical cancer. This is sexually transmitted and is the prime cause of cervical cancer in the UK. HPV immunisation is now offered to girls (aged 12 to 14) as part of the immunisation schedule to protect against cervical cancer.

Enveloped RNA viruses

Flaviviridae

Hepatitis C

This is a virus which affects the liver, with the majority of people contracting it developing a chronic disease which can lead to liver cancer or cirrhosis. It is transmitted by blood and body fluid transmission, primarily through blood rather than sexual contact. The majority of people in the UK with hepatitis C are either those who received blood transfusions prior to 1991 or intravenous drug users.

People can have the virus for several decades before developing any symptoms, particularly those who are generally fit and well. Patients with the virus do not need to be routinely isolated in hospital. NICE has a CKS for hepatitis C and also clinical guidelines for its treatment with anti-viral agents.

Coronaviridae

SARS (severe acute respiratory syndrome)

This condition was first reported in 2002 in China. It causes pyrexia, headaches, general discomfort, a dry cough and sometimes diarrhoea and can have a significant mortality rate. It is transmitted by respiratory droplets or by touching a contaminated object and then touching the mouth, nose or eyes. If admitted to hospital, patients with SARS should be isolated (see Chapter 9). SARS has not been an issue in the UK so far, but it is worth considering what occurred in China in case it does eventually cause problems worldwide. Staff caring for patients with SARS need to wear masks to protect themselves and these need to be properly fit tested so the usual paper theatre masks are not adequate for this purpose.

Retroviridae

HIV

Transmission of this virus is through blood and body fluids, mainly sexual contact, contaminated needles and mother to baby transmission. Infection with HIV is often not evident which means that a person is infectious to others without knowing that they are infected themselves. It is currently thought that all patients who are HIV positive will subsequently develop AIDS. AIDS is diagnosed when one of a list of illnesses, called AIDS defining illnesses, is diagnosed. Treatment options for HIV and AIDS are much improved and it is no longer considered to be 'a death sentence' in the way that it initially was. Patients with HIV or AIDS do not need to be routinely isolated in hospital and usual infection prevention and control precautions are enough (see Chapter 8). NICE has a CKS for HIV.

Activity 4.2 *Evidence-based practice and research*

Go online and find out what illnesses are considered to be 'AIDS defining' by the CDC (the Centers for Disease Control in America). Details of their website can be found at the end of the chapter.

Answers at the end of the chapter.

Paramyxoviridae

Measles

This infection causes pyrexia, conjunctivitis, a cough, a red blotchy skin rash and spots in the mouth known as **Koplik spots**. It can lead to complications such as pneumonia, otitis media and encephalitis. It is transmitted by airborne droplet and by direct contact with respiratory secretions. Many doctors have never seen a case of measles and it is therefore sometimes difficult to diagnose. Patients hospitalised with measles are usually isolated until they have had the rash for four days. NICE has a CKS for measles. There has been controversy in recent years due to concerns about the MMR vaccine, which protects against measles.

Case study

Following a research publication by Dr Andrew Wakefield, people in the UK were concerned about the suggested strong link between the MMR vaccination and autism, with some lesser concern about a link with serious bowel conditions. As a consequence of this, uptake of the vaccination in the UK fell and there was a rise in cases of measles and in clusters and outbreaks of the infection. Some children became seriously ill and there was public demand for children to be immunised with single vaccines rather than the combination vaccine. This was resisted in many parts of the UK as it was considered to be unnecessary. Following on from these events, Dr Wakefield's research was discredited and he was struck off by the General Medical Council. However, the consequences of his publication were longer lasting. Consider the activity below.

Activity 4.3	*Evidence-based practice and research*

In 2013 the Chief Medical Officer at the Department of Health published a letter aimed at GPs and Directors of Public Health in response to an increase in measles in some parts of the UK. Go online and access this letter via a link on the following page: **www.gov.uk/government/collections/MMR-catch-up-programme-2013**. What does it tell you about measles cases in England and Wales at the beginning of 2013 and which group is primarily affected? What are GPs advised to do?

Answers at the end of the chapter.

The vaccine discussed above also protects against mumps and rubella.

Mumps

Acute infection causes pyrexia and swelling of the salivary glands. In males it can lead to inflammation of the testes (orchitis), in females inflammation of the ovaries (oophiritis) and in both genders can result in meningitis, encephalitis, deafness, arthritis, pericarditis, arthritis and pancreatitis. It is transmitted by airborne droplets and through contact with infected respiratory secretions. If hospitalised, patients should be isolated, usually until five days after the swelling of the glands began. NICE has a CKS for mumps.

Respiratory syncytial virus (RSV)

This is a common virus in young children under the age of one year. It often causes a condition called **bronchiolitis** which has symptoms such as a runny nose, high temperature, cough, rapid or noisy breathing and difficulty feeding (Openshaw, 2010). It can also cause pneumonia.

In adults it also causes bronchitis. The virus is transmitted by respiratory droplets or by contamination on hands. It is estimated that in the UK, by the age of two most children will have been infected by RSV, with half of these having bronchiolitis as a result. Antiviral treatment is not completely effective and in hospital, cases are usually isolated and provided with symptomatic support such as oxygen therapy (see Chapters 8 and 9 for infection prevention and control precautions).

Togaviridae

Rubella

This condition results in a pinkish rash which usually begins on the face. It also causes mild pyrexia. It is generally a mild disease with few complications. However, if caught in the first trimester of pregnancy, it can cause congenital rubella which can result in spontaneous abortion, foetal death or organ damage. It is transmitted by airborne droplets and direct contact with respiratory secretions and can be protected against through the MMR vaccination. In hospital, patients should be isolated until they have had the rash for four days.

Filoviridae

Ebola

This is a viral haemorrhagic fever of the Filiviridae classification and previously it was considered to be a problem that did not fully concern the Western world. More recently, however, travellers from places such as Africa have returned with the virus and healthcare workers have become infected. It is therefore considered appropriate here to provide some basic information about the condition should a similar situation arise during your nursing programme as the issue is continuing. It might also be of use should you undertake an overseas placement or consider working in an at-risk area in the future. Ebola is considered to be a cause of viral haemorrhagic fever as it causes bleeding into the skin, the mucous membranes, organs and the gastro-intestinal tract and it also causes pyrexia (Sharts-Hopko, 2015). The mortality rate can be higher than 50%. Ebola is transmitted by the blood and body fluid route and strict standard precautions are required. In the UK, patients with Ebola are isolated in negative pressure rooms in addition to other strict precautions (see Chapter 9). As a healthcare worker you would need to adhere to these strict precautions if caring for such a patient as in later stages of the disease, all body fluids are infectious.

Activity 4.4   *Evidence-based practice and research*

Go to the Public Health England website at **www.gov.uk/government/organisations/public-health-england** and access the 'Ebola infection prevention and control guidance for primary care'. Answer the following questions:

- When individuals ring the surgery, which people should be advised NOT to visit the surgery?
- If a patient visits a GP surgery and says they may have been exposed to Ebola, what should happen next?

Answers at the end of the chapter.

Orthomyxoviridae

Influenza

Also known as flu, this causes a respiratory infection with associated pyrexia, general aches, cough and sore throat. In children it can also cause diarrhoea and vomiting. In severe cases it can lead to pneumonia and bronchitis, leading to death. There are three main types of influenza virus. Type A causes severe cases and is the type usually associated with pandemics and epidemics (Kiser and Santibanez, 2014).This is also the type which mutates each year and therefore changes, which has an impact on the annual 'flu' vaccine which needs to be changed and administered every year to those at risk. Type B is less severe and leads to more localised outbreaks. Type C usually causes very mild disease and does not cause epidemics. Influenza is spread by airborne droplets and direct contact with respiratory secretions. It has been known for flu that affects birds (avian flu) to be transferred to humans. Each year in the UK there is a flu campaign to identify and immunise those considered to be at higher risk of death from influenza. Nurses help in these campaigns by identifying those at risk and by administering and assisting with immunisations. It is worth noting here that the influenza vaccine is not a live vaccine and therefore cannot cause flu. This belief is sometimes one of the reasons for people refusing the vaccine each year. It is important they have the vaccine each year if at risk as it is based on the southern hemisphere flu virus which has been circulating and is therefore expected here each year. NICE has a CKS for influenza. There are also national guidelines for the management of patients with influenza published by organisations such as Public Health England, Public Health Wales, Health Protection Scotland and the Public Health Agency in Northern Ireland.

Activity 4.5   *Evidence-based practice and research*

Go to the Public Health England website and find out which people are at higher risk from influenza virus and therefore need to be immunised as part of the immunisation schedule each year.

The answers can be found at the end of this chapter.

Non-enveloped RNA viruses

Picornaviridae

Hepatitis A

This is transmitted by the faecal–oral route, primarily via contaminated water and shell-fish. It can cause a mild illness which lasts from one to two weeks but can also be more severe lasting several months (Matheny and Kingery, 2012). Symptoms can include jaundice, diarrhoea, general aches and tiredness, abdominal pain, joint pain and a change in urine colour. Outbreaks can be caused in settings where hand hygiene is poor such as in schools and nurseries. In the hospital setting, patients should be isolated until diarrhoea has ceased for 48 hours or until they have been jaundiced for seven days. NICE has a CKS for hepatitis A.

Calciviridae

Norovirus

This infection is transmitted by the faecal–oral route and causes nausea, vomiting and diarrhoea. It is responsible for outbreaks in hospitals, nursing and residential homes and cruise ships. It is generally self-limiting but can last longer in the elderly and in the immuno-compromised. If there are other health conditions it can also prove fatal to a small number of people (Norovirus Working Party, 2012). Patients in hospital should be isolated until they have been symptom-free for 48 hours and hand hygiene is of vital importance. Staff commonly become infected when caring for patients with the virus and when this occurs, staff should stay at home until symptom-free for 48 hours to limit spread.

Case study

According to Public Health England, there were 539 hospital outbreaks of norovirus in England in the first 32 weeks of 2015. The BBC News website reported on one of the outbreaks as follows:

An outbreak of norovirus in Cornwall has prompted the closure of four hospital wards across the county.

*The **Royal Cornwall Hospital Trust** has closed three wards in Truro and one at the West Cornwall Hospital in Penzance.*

Health bosses are urging any members of the public with norovirus symptoms of sickness or diarrhoea to stay away from hospitals and care homes.

The hospital trust has been on 'black alert' twice in 2015 due to pressure on its services.

*Natalie Jones, from **NHS Kernow**, said: 'We know some people feel under pressure to visit their loved ones in hospital or a care home, even if they're also unwell.'*

'Please consider your own health and that of other people and stay away from hospital until you're better.'

The trust asked people to avoid going to the emergency department at Royal Cornwall Hospital in Truro if they are able manage the symptoms themselves.

This case study demonstrates the consequences of outbreaks of norovirus, both in terms of ward closures and visiting ill patients when you have symptoms.

Hepatitis E

This has similar symptoms to hepatitis A and is transmitted by the faecal–oral route, usually via contaminated water (Ruggeri et al., 2013). It is rare in the UK and is usually contracted through foreign travel to countries such as India and Mexico. It is usually self-limiting but can cause chronic liver disease in the immuno-suppressed. It can cause particular problems in pregnancy. If caught in the third trimester it can cause premature labour and infant death. It can also cause maternal death due to liver failure. As there is currently no vaccination, pregnant women need to take particular care when travelling to countries where hepatitis E is common. In the UK it is most commonly transmitted through contaminated meat, so good food hygiene and proper cooking of meat is important.

Reoviridae

Rotavirus

There are seven serogroups of this virus with the most significant being group A. This is responsible for most outbreaks. It is transmitted by the faecal–oral route and causes diarrhoea and vomiting. Outbreaks occur in nurseries due to poor hand hygiene. In the hospital setting, patients should be isolated until symptom-free for 48 hours. There is usually no treatment required as the infection is self-limiting and will resolve on its own. However, the rotavirus vaccine is now part of the childhood immunisation programme in the UK.

Immunisation

Some viruses can be protected against through the use of immunisation. Vaccines work by inducing active immunity which is the term used to describe protection that is produced by a person's own immune system. This can be termed either antibody-mediated (caused by B cells) or cell-mediated (caused by T-cells). Vaccines also provide immunological memory so that the immune system can respond more quickly to exposure to an infection in the future. Vaccines can be made from a variety of products including live organisms, secretions and cell wall components.

Activity 4.6	*Evidence-based practice and research*

Go online and look at the green book 'Immunisation against infectious diseases' (website at the end of this chapter). Which viruses can be immunised against? What is the current immunisation schedule in the UK for children up to one year?

Answers at the end of the chapter.

In addition to prevention by immunisation, treatment options are available for some viral infections.

Treatment of viral infections

Many viral infections resolve without treatment but in some infections, anti-viral drugs are given to slow down viral replication. Such drugs are quite recent in their development – it is not so long ago that there was no treatment for viral infections. Antiviral drugs work by inhibiting the replication of the virus within host cells. Table 4.2 gives examples of such drugs and the infections that they are most useful for.

Antiviral drug	Virus/infection treated
Aciclovir Ganciclovir Valganciclovir	Herpes simplex infections Herpes zoster CMV
Oseltamivir Zanamivir Amantadine	Influenza
Lamivudine Indinavir Zidovudine Rilpivirine	HIV
Entecavir Telbivudine Adefovir Dipivoxil Peginterferon alfa Entecavir Tenofovir disoproxil	Hepatitis B
Peginterferon alfa Ribavirin Sofosbuvir Interferon alfa Simeprevir	Hepatitis C
Palivizumab	RSV

Table 4.2: Antiviral drugs

Specific anti-viral drugs are used in some infections such as hepatitis B, with several treatment options.

Activity 4.7 — Evidence-based practice and research

Go to the NICE website (**www.nice.org.uk**) and access the clinical guideline (CG165) about the diagnosis and management of viral hepatitis B then answer the following questions:

1. What three drugs are recommended for the treatment of chronic hepatitis B?

2. What treatment should be offered to those who are co-infected with chronic hepatitis B and C?

Answers found at the end of the chapter.

It is now time to try some multiple choice questions to assess your new knowledge from this chapter.

Activity 4.8 — *Multiple choice questions*

1. Which of the following is a non-enveloped DNA virus?

   a) HPV
   b) Smallpox
   c) Hepatitis B
   d) HIV
   e) Norovirus

2. Which group of viruses does measles belong to?

   a) Parvoviridae
   b) Hepadnaviridae
   c) Calciviridae
   d) Filoviridae
   e) Paramyxoviridae

3. Which of the following groups of viruses has a helical capsid?

   a) Parvoviridae
   b) Flaviviridae
   c) Reoviridae
   d) Hepadnaviridae
   e) Filoviridae

4. Which of the following virus groups can be subdivided in terms of polarity?

   a) Single stranded DNA viruses
   b) Single stranded RNA viruses
   c) Double stranded DNA viruses
   d) Double stranded RNA viruses
   e) Triple stranded RNA viruses

5. For which of the following viruses is there not an immunisation in the UK?

   a) Measles
   b) Mumps
   c) CMV
   d) Varicella zoster
   e) Influenza

6. Which of the following antiviral drugs is commonly used for herpes infections?

   a) Peginterferon alfa
   b) Zidovudine
   c) Aciclovir

(Continued)

continued . . .

    d)   Zanamivir

    e)   Ribavirin

Hopefully this activity has enabled you to test what you have gained from this chapter in terms of knowledge about viruses.

Answers provided at the end of the chapter.

Chapter summary

This chapter has introduced you to viral classification and some of the more common viruses that you will come across in healthcare. The table presented within it also details other viruses which are not covered in this chapter. We have also looked at some of the interventions in terms of immunisation and anti-viral treatments which are available in the UK. You should now have an increased knowledge and awareness of viruses which cause infection in humans.

Activities: Brief outline answers

Activity 4.2: Evidence-based practice and research (page 64)

Go online and find out what illnesses are considered to be 'AIDS defining'.

- Bacterial infections, multiple or recurrent (in children younger than 13)
- Candidiasis of bronchi, trachea, or lungs
- Candidiasis of oesophagus
- Cervical cancer, invasive (among those older than 13)
- Coccidioidomycosis, disseminated or extrapulmonary
- Cryptococcosis, extrapulmonary
- Cryptosporidiosis, chronic intestinal (>1 month's duration)
- Cytomegalovirus disease (other than liver, spleen, or nodes), onset at age >1 month
- Cytomegalovirus retinitis (with loss of vision)
- Encephalopathy, HIV related
- Herpes simplex: chronic ulcers (>1 month's duration) or bronchitis, pneumonitis, or esophagitis (onset at age >1 month)
- Histoplasmosis, disseminated or extrapulmonary
- Isosporiasis, chronic intestinal (>1 month's duration)
- Kaposi sarcoma
- Lymphoid interstitial pneumonia or pulmonary lymphoid hyperplasia complex (in those younger than 13)
- Lymphoma, Burkitt (or equivalent term)
- Lymphoma, immunoblastic (or equivalent term)
- Lymphoma, primary, of brain
- *Mycobacterium avium* complex or *Mycobacterium kansasii*, disseminated or extrapulmonary
- *Mycobacterium tuberculosis* of any site, pulmonary (in those over 13), disseminated, or extrapulmonary
- *Mycobacterium*, other species or unidentified species, disseminated or extrapulmonary

- *Pneumocystis jirovecii* pneumonia
- Pneumonia, recurrent (in over 13s)
- Progressive multifocal leukoencephalopathy
- *Salmonella* septicaemia, recurrent
- Toxoplasmosis of brain, onset at age >1 month
- Wasting syndrome attributed to HIV

Activity 4.3: Evidence-based practice and research (page 65)

Consider recent issues with vaccine uptake in relation to MMR and the resulting increase in measles in some areas of the UK. This was due to a paper published by Dr Andrew Wakefield which has since been discredited. In 2013 the Chief Medical Officer at the Department of Health published a letter aimed at GPs and Directors of Public Health. Go online and access this letter via a link on the following page: **www.gov.uk/government/collections/MMR-catch-up-programme-2013**. What does it tell you about measles cases in England and Wales at the beginning of 2013 and which group is primarily affected? What are GPs advised to do?

There have been outbreaks in Wales and an increase in incidence in the first three months of 2013, primarily in the age group which may have missed MMR immunisation due to the controversy and concern.

GPs are advised to identify those who need vaccinating and ensure they have stocks of the MMR vaccine on-site.

Activity 4.4: Evidence-based practice and research (page 66)

Go to the Public Health England website and access the 'Ebola infection prevention and control guidance for primary care'. Answer the following questions:

- When individuals ring the surgery, which people should be advised NOT to visit the surgery?
  Those who have visited an affected country within the last 21 days and are unwell and/or who report a temperature >37.5° or a history of fever within the past 24 hours.
- If a patient visits a GP surgery and says they may have been exposed to Ebola, what should happen next?
  Isolate immediately in a single, minimally furnished room, assess without physical contact; if patient has visited an affected area in the past 21 days and is unwell and has a fever or has had a fever within the last 24 hours, advice should be sought from the local microbiologist, virologist or infectious diseases doctor. Depending on advice from these, the patient may need to be transferred to the local A&E department.

Activity 4.5: Evidence-based practice and research (page 67)

Go to the Public Health England website and find out which people are at higher risk from influenza virus and therefore need to be immunised as part of the immunisation schedule each year.

- older people
- the very young
- pregnant women
- those with underlying disease, particularly chronic respiratory or cardiac disease
- those who are immuno-suppressed.

Activity 4.6: Evidence-based practice and research (page 69)

Go online and look at the green book 'Immunisation against infectious diseases' (website address at the end of this chapter). Which of the viruses can be immunised against?

Answer: hepatitis A, hepatitis B, HPV, influenza, measles, mumps, polio, rubella, Varicella zoster, RSV, rotavirus.

What is the current immunisation schedule in the UK for children up to one year?

- *Age 2 months – DPT, polio & Hib in 1 injection plus PCV in 1 injection, rotavirus orally.*
- *Age 3 months – DPT, polio & Hib in 1 injection, plus MenC in 1 injection, rotavirus orally.*
- *Age 4 months – DPT, polio & Hib in 1 injection plus MenC in 1 injection & PCV in 1 injection.*

Activity 4.7: Evidence-based practice and research (page 70)

Go to the NICE website (**www.nice.org.uk**) and access the clinical guideline (CG165) about the diagnosis and management of viral hepatitis B then answer the following questions:

1. What three drugs are recommended for the treatment of chronic hepatitis B?

Answer: Peginterferon alfa-2a, Entecavir and Tenofovir disoproxil.

2. What treatment should be offered to those who are co-infected with chronic hepatitis B and C?

Answer: peginterferon alfa and ribavirin.

Activity 4.8: MCQs (pages 71–2)

1. Which of the following is a non-enveloped DNA virus?

    a) HPV

2. Which group of viruses does measles belong to?

    e) Paramyxoviridae

3. Which of the following groups of viruses has a helical capsid?

    e) Filoviridae

4. Which of the following virus groups can be subdivided in terms of polarity?

    b) Single stranded RNA viruses

5. For which of the following viruses is there not an immunisation in the UK?

    c) CMV

6. Which of the following antiviral drugs is commonly used for herpes infections?

    c) Aciclovir

Further reading

Carter, J and Saunders, V (2013) *Virology: Principles and Applications*, 2nd edition. Oxford: John Wiley & Sons.

This book provides more in-depth information about viruses for students with a specific interest in this sub-group of micro-organisms.

Crawford, DH (2011) *Viruses: A Very Short Introduction*. Oxford: Oxford University Press.

This is a very simple, easy to understand text book covering viruses including information about the global consequences of viral infections.

Harvey, RA and Nau Cornelissen, C (2012) *Lippincott's Illustrated Reviews: Microbiology*, 3rd edition. Philadelphia: Lippincott Williams & Wilkins.

This book provides an easy to understand section on viruses and covers additional viruses not discussed in this text book.

Health Protection Agency (2011) *Viral rash in pregnancy*. London: HPA. Available at: www.gov.uk/government/uploads/system/uploads/attachment_data/file/322688/Viral_rash_in_pregnancy_guidance.pdf

NICE (2012) *Hepatitis B and C: ways to promote and offer testing to people at increased risk of infection*. London: NICE.

This document considers the ways in which healthcare professionals can increase testing in groups at risk of hepatitis B and C such as intravenous drug users.

Public Health England (2012) *Guidelines for the management of norovirus outbreaks in acute and community health and social care settings.* London: PHE.

These guidelines are relevant in both acute and primary care in relation to outbreaks in places such as hospitals, schools, nursing and residential homes etc.

Public Health England (2014) *Guidance on infection control in schools and other childcare settings.* London: PHE.

This document provides information on different infections in schools and advice on exclusions, precautions etc. including viral infections.

Useful websites

www.gov.uk/government/organisations/public-health-england

Public Health England – various guidelines and information sources are available via this site in relation to viral infections.

www.britishlivertrust.org.uk

The British Liver Trust website contains lots of information about viruses which affect the liver, in particular viral hepatitis.

www.gov.uk/government/collections/immunisation-against-infectious-disease-the-green-book

Referred to earlier in this chapter, this site provides the most up-to-date information about vaccinations offered in the UK and is updated when new vaccines are developed or added to the national immunisation schedule. This source (the green book) is referred to in Activity 4.6.

www.cdc.gov

Referred to earlier in the chapter, this is the website for the Centers for Disease Control in America.

http://cks.nice.org.uk

This website links to the Clinical Knowledge Summaries produced by NICE and referred to earlier in the chapter.

www.gov.uk/government/collections/seasonal-influenza-guidance-data-and-analysis#management-and-treatment

This website links to the PHE page for influenza information.

Chapter 5
Fungi, parasites and prions

Chapter aims

After reading this chapter, you will be able to:

*   Identify some of the fungi and parasites of significance to nursing practice.
*   Understand what prions are and what their implications are for infection prevention and control.
*   Discuss some of the treatment options for fungi and parasites.

This chapter covers three main topics: fungi, parasites and prions. We will first consider fungi in terms of their classification and some of the fungal infections of note in healthcare. Following this we will look at parasitic classifications, again looking at some of the important parasites that nurses might see in practice. The chapter concludes by looking at prions, the diseases that they cause, and their significance in healthcare. Throughout the chapter are activities and scenarios to enable you to both gain more knowledge and to test your knowledge.

People with no worms in their gut are in the minority! More than three-quarters of people in the world have a worm of some kind in their gut, whether it be very small, or several feet long!
(Maxmen, 2009)

Fungi

Of the more than 100,000 species of known fungi, less than 500 cause disease in humans, with the majority of these causing problems for immuno-compromised individuals (Brown et al., 2012). Some infections are caused by fungi from the environment whereas others are caused by endogenous fungi which can be opportunistic in nature. Fungi cause diseases which are sometimes referred to as mycoses.

There are several different ways of classifying fungi. They can be considered to be superficial, subcutaneous, deep or systemic, for example. For the purposes of this chapter, we will consider three categories: yeast or yeast-like, filamentous and dimorphic.

Yeast/yeast-like

These are considered to be similar to bacteria in that they exist as single spherical cells which are not connected. Unlike bacteria, however, they can be up to ten times larger. This type of fungus generally reproduces using a process known as **budding**. Fungi in this group include *Candida albicans, Cryptococcus neoformans* and *Pneumocystis jiroveci.*

Candida albicans

This fungus is part of the normal flora in various parts of the body including the gastro-intestinal tract. It is also commonly found in the mouth and the female genital tract. It can cause both superficial and more serious infections. The one that most people are aware of is vaginal thrush which women commonly get following antibiotics where the flora of the genital tract is disturbed, or with the use of some products such as bubble bath. Oral candida infections are also fairly common. Such superficial infections are often treated with oral suspensions such as nystatin or topical ointments/**pessaries** such as clotrimazole. More serious infections can occur in the gastro-intestinal tract, lungs and urinary tract and even in the brain. Consider the case study below.

Case study

Dorothy is a 58-year-old woman admitted for a routine eye operation. Unfortunately, during her operation she has a cardiac arrest. Following resuscitation she is ventilated with a machine to help

(Continued)

continued . . .

her to breathe on intensive care where she also has invasive devices including a urinary catheter, a central line and peripheral intravenous devices which are both lines to access veins to provide fluids and medicines. Her eye and one peripheral line become infected with Candida albicans. Her condition later improves and she is taken off the ventilator and is transferred to a medical ward for recovery. When on this ward she becomes confused and has headaches. Further investigations indicate that the Candida albicans infection has now travelled to the brain – she now has candida of the brain, a life-threatening infection. She is treated with intravenous anti-fungal drugs including amphotericin but subsequently dies from her infection.

The above case study demonstrates that patients can die from fungal infections. In particular, *Candida albicans* infections are considered by many to be minor and easily treated – this case study highlights the potential severity of the infection if it affects areas such as the brain.

Where candida infections are more serious, such as in the case above, the previous-mentioned treatments are of limited value. Medications such as fluconazole, polyenes and echinocandins (see Table 5.1 later in the chapter) may therefore be required. There are side effects to these medications, some of which can be severe.

Cryptococcus neoformans

This fungus is commonly found in pigeon faeces and when inhaled can cause lung infections which can pass into both the bloodstream and the cerebro-spinal fluid. This can all lead to pulmonary disease, meningitis or more widespread disease where more than one area of the body is affected. The most common form of infection is a mild lung infection but if this disseminates, which is often the case in immuno-compromised patients, it can be fatal. The fungus is not spread from person to person and patients infected with it therefore do not need to be isolated. Standard infection control precautions apply. Cryptococcus infections can be treated with drugs such as fluconazole, amphotericin and flucytosine.

Pneumocystis jiroveci (formerly known as Pneumocystis carinii)

Infection with this fungus used to be rare but immuno-suppression related to the use of some medications and AIDS has led to an increase in cases, usually causing pneumonia. In those whose immune systems are functioning correctly it causes asymptomatic infection but in the immuno-compromised it can cause pyrexia, breathing difficulties, cough and cyanosis. It can be fatal if left untreated. Patients do not usually need to be isolated but standard infection prevention and control precautions apply. The route of transmission is currently unclear but may be by direct contact or contact with respiratory secretions (droplet spread). Previously this fungus was considered to be protozoal in nature. Treatment recommended in the UK is co-trimoxazole, which is a combination of two drugs: trimethoprim and sulfathoxazole.

Filamentous

This type of fungi are also known as mould-like. The body of this type is generally a collection of threads with multiple branches. These threads grow by either branching or lengthening their tips. The threads are known as hyphae. Fungi within this group include *Aspergillus fumigatus* and dermatophytes.

Aspergillus fumigatus

This fungus can be found in soil and has been cultured from air and water. Outbreaks have occurred in hospital where the fungus has been dispersed during building work. People become infected with this organism through inhalation or via the gastro-intestinal tract. It generally causes lung disease such as pneumonia but can spread from there to the bloodstream, liver, kidneys and brain. Those who become infected are usually those who are **neutropenic**, on corticosteroids, on other immuno-suppressive drugs or who are transplant recipients. Invasive infection does not generally occur in those with a competent immune system. Pulmonary infections cause symptoms such as pyrexia, chest pain, cough, **dyspnoea** and **haemoptysis**. Where the infection has spread beyond the lungs there can be necrotic skin lesions and brain abscesses, the latter leading to strokes or seizures. Prevention in high-risk areas of the hospital can be assisted by providing filtered air, minimising exposure to dust from construction work and discouraging high-risk patients from participating in activities such as building work. Patients do not need to be isolated to prevent the spread of this infection but standard precautions should be applied. However, patients who become severely neutropenic may need to be isolated for their own protection (see Chapter 9). *Aspergillus* infections can be treated with echinocandins and amphotericin.

Dermatophytes

These fungi affect the skin and related structures and are sometimes referred to as dermatophytosis or tinea. Transmission from one person to another is by infected skin scales. Dermatophytes use keratin as their nutrition source which means that they can infect structures with keratin in them such as the skin, hair and nails. Dermatophytes are transmitted by direct or indirect contact with lesions. Some infections cause mildly irritating skin scaling and redness but sometimes there can be itching, swelling, blisters and more severe skin scaling. Dermatophyte infections are commonly treated with topical creams and ointments such as those in the imidazole group of anti-fungal agents. There are three important types:

1. *Epidermophyton* – infects skin (Tinea corporis, also known as ringworm), nails (Tinea unguium, also known as onchymycosis), groin (Tinea cruris, commonly referred to as 'jock itch') and feet (Tinea pedis, also known as athlete's foot). This type of dermatophyte does not infect hair. Where nails are infected, oral treatment can include terbafine. This can also be used for ringworm if oral rather than topical treatment is required.

2. *Microsporum* – infects the scalp, often referred to as ringworm of the scalp. This condition can also be caused by trichophyton. The type of dermatophyte causing the scalp infection tends to be dependent on the country of infection.

3. *Trichophyton* – infects the feet, nails and groin. In children, an anti-fungal agent called griseofulvin may be used.

Patients infected with dermatophytes do not generally need to be admitted to hospital and will most commonly be treated in primary care via the GP.

Dimorphic

Fungi which are yeast-like in one environment and mould-like in another are referred to as dimorphic. Aspects such as temperature and carbon dioxide level can change the way that the fungus behaves. *Histoplasma capsulatum* and *Blastomyces dermatidis* belong in this fungal group.

Histoplasma capsulatum

This can be found in soil, bird and bat droppings and can enter the respiratory tract through inhalation. It is not usually transmitted from person to person. Patients can be asymptomatic but can also have acute or chronic disease, with symptoms including pyrexia, headache and lethargy. Chronic disease tends to affect those with pre-existing lung conditions. Patients do not need to be isolated and standard infection control precautions apply. Infection does not always need treating but if symptoms persist it can be treated with itraconazole or, if more severe, amphotericin.

Blastomyces dermatidis

This is a soil mould which becomes a yeast after it is inhaled. It is not usually transmitted from person to person. It causes skin lesions, pulmonary disease and sometimes a more widespread infection. Initially the fungus is inhaled, entering the lungs and causing a pulmonary infection. It is rare for this initial infection to spread to other sites but when it does it can infect the skin, bones and genito-urinary tract. Patients with the infection do not need to be isolated in hospital. Infection can be treated with triazoles or imidazoles.

While many patients with fungal infections do not require hospitalisation, as nurses we may be required to give advice and information about such infections in primary care settings.

Activity 5.1   *Evidence-based practice and research*

Consider the following three fungal infections. If you were in contact with a patient, either in the primary care or hospital setting, with each of these infections, what do you think they need to know about their condition? Go online and find out further information about these infections for your answers.

- Tinea pedis
- *Candida albicans* of the mouth
- *Aspergillus fumigatus* lung infection in a neutropenic patient

Suggested answers can be found at the end of this chapter.

You will have found from this activity that there is a lot of information available for both nurses and their patients which we can utilise in managing and preventing the spread of their infections.

Fungal diseases can also be classified in terms of how serious the disease is and the type of fungus causing it. Five general classifications can be used:

1. Superficial mycoses.

2. **Subcutaneous** mycoses.

3. Deep mycoses caused by opportunistic pathogens.

4. **Systemic** mycoses caused by opportunistic pathogens.

5. Systemic mycoses caused by primary pathogens.

Fungi can be classified within several of these groups depending on the disease that they cause. For example, *Candida albicans* can cause several of these types of mycoses. These classifications are important in healthcare as they signify how serious the infection is, who is at risk and where the cause has come from.

The treatment of fungal infections

Treatment can be with topical creams or ointments, oral medication or intravenous medication. Table 5.1 gives examples of treatments offered in the UK. It would be beneficial to familiarise yourself with some of these so that if patients tell you that they are taking these medications, you have some idea why they are taking them.

Drug group	Drug names
Triazoles	Fluconazole
	Itraconazole
	Posaconazole
	Voriconazole
Imidazoles	Clotrimazole
	Econazole
	Ketoconazole
	Tioconazole
Polyenes	Amphotericin
	Nystatin
Echinocandins	Anidulafungin
	Caspofungin
	Micofungin
Others	Flucytosine
	Griseofulvin
	Terbafine

Table 5.1: Treatments for fungal infections

Further information about different fungal infections and their current recommended treatments in the UK can be gained from the British National Formulary. This is available in practice areas as a book or online via the website **www.medicinescomplete.com/mc/bnf/current** for adults and **www.medicinescomplete.com/mc/bnfc/current** for children.

Parasites

Parasites can be considered to be types of worm (helminths), types of insects (ectoparasites) or protozoa.

Worms (helminths)

Thread worms

These are small worms which infect the large intestine and lay eggs around the anus. They cause itching in the anal and vaginal areas – this is caused by them secreting mucous. The itching can be worse at night. It can be transmitted by the hands following scratching and other people can then become infected. It is a relatively mild condition which can be treated with mebendazole – when a person is found to be infected, their whole household should usually be treated and good hand hygiene is important. This condition is usually managed in the community.

Tape worms

These worms also infect the large intestine but unlike the smaller threadworm, can grow as long as 9 metres. They are transmitted by the faecal–oral route and can be ingested in contaminated food. Often there are no symptoms but some people can experience abdominal pain, diarrhoea and vomiting. Treatment only kills the worm and not any eggs that it has laid, so hygiene is very important. Some people notice segments of the worm in their faeces when they go to the toilet. Depending on the type of tapeworm causing the infection, treatment can be complicated and while most people are managed in the community, some may require surgery to remove the worm. If admitted to hospital due to complications caused by either thread or tape worms, standard precautions apply (see Chapter 8).

Ectoparasites

Head lice

These are tiny insects that infect the scalp. They are transmitted by direct head to head contact so they do not fly, jump or swim. They do not discriminate between clean and dirty hair so anyone can be infected. When living moving lice are found in the hair, treatment should be commenced. Other people should then be checked such as friends and family members. Those found to have living moving lice should also be treated. While it is considered a childhood problem, it can infect people of any age. It is managed in the community, but can cause a lot of concern for parents with children at school. It can also cause outbreaks in long-term care settings such as nursing and residential homes. Treatment can be by lotions, sprays or a technique called wet combing where a special comb is used to drag the lice from the hair. Treatments include malathion and permethrin.

As can be seen from the scenario above, head lice is not just an infection of children, and adults should therefore be checked as contacts if children are found to be infected (including parents and grandparents).

Scabies

This is a skin condition caused by a mite known as *Sarcoptes scabiei* which burrows under the skin. Its excretions and secretions cause itching and a rash which is not related to the location of the mites in the body. There are two main types of scabies: classical and Norwegian. The latter tends to affect people who are immuno-compromised most often. Scabies is transmitted by prolonged skin-to-skin contact, and can be treated with lotions called malathion or permethrin. Again, this parasite is usually managed in the community unless the rash becomes infected when hospital treatment may be recommended for some people. Standard infection prevention and control precautions should be applied (Chapter 8) but isolation is not generally required.

Protozoa

These are unicellular organisms and only a few of the tens of thousands of species are pathogenic to humans. These tend to affect either the intestinal/urogenital tracts or the blood and tissues. Protozoal diseases are most common in developing tropical and sub-tropical regions but foreign travel and immigration mean that, as nurses in the UK, we will inevitably come across such conditions. Major protozoa are generally classified into four main groups: ciliates; amoebae; flagellates and sporozoa. Some of the protozoa in these groups will now be considered in more detail. Some protozoal infections are notifiable which you will remember was discussed in Chapter 1.

Giardia lamblia

This is a flagellate which affects the intestinal tract. The parasite generally inhabits the duodenum which means that if a stool sample is examined it may be negative. Infections with this parasite are generally mild but some patients can have damage to their duodenal mucosa. Its main symptom is diarrhoea but it can also cause abdominal cramps, nausea, bloating, fatigue, loss of appetite and weight loss. It is commonly treated with metronidazole, but often symptoms resolve within a week and treatment is not required. In the hospital setting, patients with diarrhoea are commonly isolated until they have been symptom-free for 48 hours to minimise the risk of transmission to other patients.

Cryptosporidium parvum

This is a sporozoan which affects the intestinal tract, causing diarrhoea. It is usually short-lived, but can be more severe in children and immuno-compromised individuals. It can be transmitted by contaminated food or water and may be linked in some areas to poor hygiene and sanitation. It is a common cause of diarrhoea in HIV-positive patients, and in hospital it is common for tap water to be boiled then cooled to drink in immuno-compromised patients, though this is not just in relation to *Cryptosporidium*. As a gastro-intestinal illness, this is notifiable.

Trichomonas vaginalis

This is a flagellate which affects the urogenital tract. It can cause symptoms such as inflammation and a yellow (female) or white (male) discharge, though around half of those infected will have no symptoms at all. It is primarily sexually transmitted. Complications are rare, but if caught in pregnancy it can cause premature delivery or low birth weight. It is primarily managed in primary care and treated with metronidazole.

Plasmodium species

This is a sporozoan which affects the blood and organs. This group causes different types of malaria through bites from mosquitoes. These include *Plasmodium falciparum*, *Plasmodium vivax* and *Plasmodium ovale*. Transmission can also be via blood transfusion or sharing needles, but this is very rare. Symptoms include pyrexia, fatigue, vomiting, diarrhoea and headaches. Some are more serious than others and can cause death without prompt treatment. When patients are admitted to hospital in the UK with a pyrexia of an unknown cause, questions will be asked about foreign travel and if they have travelled to an at-risk country they will be tested for malaria. Malaria is currently not acquired in the UK, but people return from travel with the condition and are treated here following holidays etc. Taking prophylaxis while in at-risk areas such as Africa and parts of Asia will protect against the condition but compliance can be poor here, resulting in infection. Treatment varies depending on the type of plasmodium species involved (see Table 5.2). Standard precautions apply (Chapter 8), but patients generally do not require isolation. However, there are some instances where patients are admitted with what is termed a 'pyrexia of unknown origin' or PUO and malaria may be suspected. In such cases, isolation (Chapter 9) may be recommended until the cause is confirmed, in case the pyrexia is caused by an infection which requires isolation.

Toxoplasma gondii

This is a sporozoan. It causes a condition known as toxoplasmosis and many people are unaware they have it due to symptoms being so mild and similar to flu. However, it can cause problems in pregnancy such as miscarriage and stillbirth. It can also cause problems in newborns who have acquired it congenitally in whom it can cause conditions such as hydrocephalus, cerebral palsy, visual defects and epilepsy; and in immuno-compromised individuals such as those with HIV who can develop encephalitis. It is commonly transmitted from cat faeces. Infection can therefore occur by consuming food, water or soil that is contaminated with infected cat's faeces. It can also be caused by eating or handling raw, undercooked infected meat, using knives and other utensils that have been in contact with undercooked or raw infected meat or drinking unpasteurised goat's milk or eating products made from it, such as cheese. Treatment is generally only required by people with compromised immune systems and these patients may be given pyrimethamine plus sulfadiazine or azithromycin. Some patients may require hospital admission for their treatment and for symptom management and standard precautions would be applied (Chapter 8).

Treatment of protozoal infections

Group	Drug examples
Antimalarials	Chloroquine Mefloquine Piperaquine Primaquine Proguanil Pyramethamine Quinine Tetracyclines
Amoebicides	Diloxanide furoate Metronidazole Tinidazole
Trichomonacides	Metronidazole Tinidazole
Antigiardials	Metronidazole Tinidazole Mepacrine hydrochloride
Leishmaniacides	Sodium stibogluconate Amphotericin Pentamidine isethionate
Trypanocides	Strain dependent
Toxoplasmosis drugs	Pyrimethamine Sulfadiazide

Table 5.2: Groups of antiprotozoal drugs

Prions

Prions are not actually micro-organisms if we wish to be completely accurate, but they can cause infection. Prions are small infectious particles made up of abnormally folded protein (normal body proteins fold abnormally and affect function). They cause progressive neurodegenerative conditions referred to as transmissible spongiform encephalopathies (TSEs) in humans. These misfolded proteins do not behave like bacteria which multiply in the host organism that they infect. Instead they affect the structure of the brain by behaving like a template, inducing proteins with normal folding to convert to the abnormal prion form. The damage caused to the brain is irreversible. They can affect humans and cause a variety of conditions including Creutzfeldt–Jakob disease (CJD), new variant vCJD (which is thought to have come from bovine spongiform encephalopathy (BSE) in cows), Kuru, fatal familial insomnia and Gerstmann–Sträussler–Scheinker syndrome (GSS). You are most likely to be familiar with CJD and vCJD as this was discussed a lot in the media after vCJD in humans was thought to have been transmitted from infected cows via the food chain in the UK. vCJD only occurs in about 1% of all CJD cases (Diack et al., 2014).

CJD

This prion disease causes symptoms such as memory loss, changes in intellect and personality, loss of balance and coordination, visual disturbances, slurred speech, jerking movements and progressive loss of mobility. It is currently thought that most people die within one year of symptoms beginning. Unfortunately, some of the initial symptoms are similar to other conditions such as dementia, and CJD may therefore not be suspected until late in the disease process or even after death. There is currently no cure for CJD, and no test that can be carried out in the UK to identify the abnormal prions in the body. There are three categories of CJD: sporadic, familial and iatrogenic, but generally they are all referred to as CJD.

Activity 5.2   *Evidence-based practice and research*

Go to the NHS Choices website and find out about each of the three categories of CJD.

Further information can be found at the end of this chapter.

Hopefully the simple information found on the NHS Choices website will have enabled you to understand the CJD categories a little more clearly in terms of who they affect and how they are acquired.

As there is no simple and easy test for CJD while a patient is alive, diagnosis is generally based on symptoms and past history, though a brain biopsy can be performed. Often, the diagnosis is confirmed by examination of the brain after death. Patients may have acquired an abnormal prion, but until it begins to have a negative effect on the brain, which may be after several years, a brain biopsy is of no value. There are, however, some tests which can indicate a strong possibility of CJD once symptoms have begun such as a lumbar puncture, MRI scan, EEG or prototype blood test (vCJD only). However, as there is no treatment for CJD, the undertaking of tests may not necessarily be of benefit to patients unless we are trying to rule out CJD to confirm another treatable condition or consider issues of decontamination of surgical instruments, for example. Consider the following scenario.

Scenario

A recently deceased patient is identified as having died from vCJD. Three months prior to his death he had surgery on his spine at the local teaching hospital. This means that patients operated on subsequently with the instruments used in his surgery may have been exposed to the infection. The instruments are identified and destroyed, but the hospital now needs to identify all patients operated on with this set of instruments since the deceased man's surgery. Because of track and trace systems within the hospital and bar coding of instruments, a list of patients is produced. There is no test for vCJD and no treatment for those exposed. There is therefore no test or treatment that can be offered to the patients on this list. Each of these patients is now at home and their GPs are informed by the hospital of their possible exposure to vCJD.

Activity 5.3   *Reflection*

Consider that you were a patient on the list in the above scenario. Would you want to be informed by your GP that you may have been exposed to vCJD, knowing there was no test that could identify whether you were infected and no treatment to be offered to you?

There is no answer for this activity.

As you might have considered, this is a difficult issue which we sometimes have to deal with in healthcare, providing patients with information, but knowing there is currently no treatment or cure that we can provide them with.

The main issue related to CJD and other prion diseases in healthcare is that they cannot be destroyed by the usual methods of decontamination such as disinfection and sterilisation. This has implications for the use of surgical instruments. Currently in healthcare we assign risks to specific tissues within the body and to different surgical procedures so that the brain and spinal cord, for example, would be considered high-risk tissues for prions. We also perform risk assessments in some areas on patients to identify those at higher risk of having an abnormal prion. These include those receiving certain procedures in the past or who have had a member of their family die from a prion disease. From an infection prevention perspective, patients with CJD do not need to be isolated and normal standard precautions apply, but it may be easier in some areas to isolate these patients to more safely manage decontamination issues (see Chapter 8). Steps have been taken to minimise the risk of CJD from food supply (e.g. cows) and from blood transfusions, the latter after a small number of cases of CJD were probably acquired via transfusion.

Fatal familial insomnia (FFI)

This is a very rare prion disease which involves insomnia which becomes worse. This then leads to symptoms such as hallucinations, delirium and confusion. All patients diagnosed with this condition have subsequently died. Genetic testing can be undertaken to see if the FFI gene is being carried, but it is estimated that less than 30 families in the world carry the gene.

It is now the time within this chapter to assess what you have gained in terms of knowledge through your reading and activities.

Activity 5.4   *Multiple choice questions*

1. Which of the following fungal infections is dimorphic in nature?

    a) *Candida albicans*
    b) *Aspergillus*
    c) *Histoplasma capsulatum*
    d) *Cryptococcus neoformans*
    e) *Tinea corporis*

2. Which of the following is a protozoon?

    a) *Sarcoptes scabiei*
    b) *Candida albicans*
    c) *Tinea capitis*
    d) *Plasmodium vivax*
    e) FFI

3. What is a prion?

    a) A bacterium
    b) A virus
    c) A fungus
    d) A parasite
    e) A protein

4. Which of the following drugs might be used to treat *Plasmodium* species?

    a) Chloroquine
    b) Metronidazole
    c) Alphoteracin
    d) Sulfadiazide
    e) Clotrimazole

5. Which of the following is a dermatophyte?

    a) *Aspergillus fumigatus*
    b) Tinea pedis

c) *Candida albicans*

d) *Histoplasma capsulatum*

e) *Cryptosporidium parvum*

6. Which of the following is NOT a prion disease?

a) Fatal familial insomnia

b) New variant CJD

c) Tinea capitis

d) CJD

e) GSS

Chapter summary

This chapter has introduced you to some of the infections caused by fungi, parasites and prions. It has also provided you with information about treatment options available for these infections and highlighted some of the infection prevention and control issues which will be discussed in more depth in Chapters 8 and 9. You should now have a better understanding of the impact of such infections on both patients and healthcare.

Activities: Brief outline answers

Activity 5.1: Evidence-based practice and research (page 80)

Consider the following three fungal infections. If you were in contact with a patient, either in the primary care or hospital setting, with each of these infections, what do you think they needed to know about their condition? You are advised to go online and find out further information about these infections for your answers.

- Tinea pedis – patients might want to know how they caught it, how to treat it, how to stop it spreading to others, how long symptoms might persist and if they might get it again.
- *Candida albicans* of the mouth – as above.
- *Aspergillus fumigatus* lung infection in a neutropenic patient – as above. In addition, patients might want to know whether their neutropenic condition will affect the outcome of the infection or vice versa, if there are any serious risks to them associated with the infection and how long it might take for the infection to be completely treated.

Activity 5.2: Evidence-based practice and research (page 86)

Go to the NHS Choices website and find out about each of the three categories of CJD.

Sporadic CJD

- The most common type of CJD.
- Suggested that in some people a normal brain protein undergoes an abnormal change (misfolding) and turns into a prion.
- Most cases occur in older adults aged between 45 and 75 years
- Very rare, affecting only 1–2 in every million people each year in the UK.

Inherited/familial CJD

- A very rare genetic condition.
- One of the genes a person inherits from their parent carries a mutation.
- It affects about 1 in every 9 million people in the UK.
- Symptoms usually first develop in people aged in their early 50s.

Iatrogenic CJD

- The infection is accidentally spread from someone with CJD through medical or surgical treatment.
- A common cause of iatrogenic CJD in the past was growth hormone treatment using human pituitary growth hormones extracted from deceased individuals, some of whom were infected with CJD. Synthetic versions of growth hormones are now used, so this is no longer a risk.
- Can also occur if instruments used during brain surgery on a person with CJD are not properly decontaminated between each surgical procedure before re-use on another person.
- Iatrogenic CJD is now very rare.

Activity 5.4: MCQs (pages 88–9)

1. Which of the following fungal infections is dimorphic in nature?

   c) *Histoplasma capsulatum*

2. Which of the following is a protozoon?

   d) *Plasmodium vivax*

3. What is a prion?

   e) A protein

4. Which of the following drugs might be used to treat *Plasmodium* species?

   a) Chloroquine

5. Which of the following is a dermatophyte?

   b) Tinea pedis

6. Which of the following is NOT a prion disease?

   c) Tinea capitis

Further reading

Richardson, MD and Warnock, DW (2012) *Fungal Infections: Diagnosis and Management,* 4th edition. Oxford: Wiley-Blackwell.

This text offers in-depth information about fungal diseases.

Zou, WQ and Gambetti, P (2012) *Prions and Diseases. Volume 1: Physiology and Pathophysiology.* New York: Springer.

This book would be suitable for students with a specific interest in prion diseases. It is very comprehensive and might be useful for projects and assignments related to the topic.

Useful websites

www.gov.uk/fungal-infections

Public Health England's page with further England related information about fungal infections.

www.gov.uk/government/collections/creutzfeldt-jakob-disease-cjd-guidance-data-and-analysis

Public Health England's page about CJD.

www.gov.uk/government/collections/malaria-guidance-data-and-analysis

Public Health England's page about malaria.

www.gov.uk/government/uploads/system/uploads/attachment_data/file/271414/Frequently_asked_questions.pdf

Frequently asked questions about prion diseases.

www.gov.uk/government/publications/guidance-from-the-acdp-tse-risk-management-subgroup-formerly-tse-working-group

Healthcare related guidance for prion diseases.

www.who.int/mediacentre/factsheets/fs180/en/

Information about vCJD from the World Health Organization.

Chapter 6
Microbiological specimens

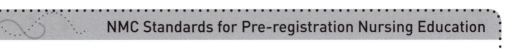
Chapter aims

After reading this chapter, you will be able to:

- Identify some of the microbiological specimens that nurses obtain and the reasons for obtaining them.
- Describe the most effective way of obtaining some of these specimens.
- Identify some of the issues relating to specimen collection in primary care settings.

Within this chapter we will look at specimens obtained and tested in healthcare to confirm whether a patient has an infection and identify treatment options. Firstly we will look at reasons for obtaining microbiological samples from patients before going on to look at different specimens that can be collected and how this should be done, including appropriate documentation. At the end of the chapter we will briefly look at some of the issues relating to specimen collection and transportation for nurses. Throughout the chapter are activities to help you to gain a wider knowledge and understanding of the subject.

In Chapter 2 we looked at some of the signs and symptoms of infection. As you may remember, some of these are very general, such as tachycardia, and may indicate something other than an infection. It is therefore important that infection is confirmed through other means such as microbiological testing. This helps to identify what organism is causing the infection and what treatments can be used. Symptoms and specimen results should be combined to decide on the best management for the patient. Similar to how signs and symptoms do not definitely confirm infection, a positive microbiological specimen result only confirms the presence of a micro-organism, not that it is causing infection. It may, for example, be part of the normal flora or be colonising the area, causing no damage. This again then stresses the importance of combining both signs and symptoms and specimen results to decide if the patient has an infection, what organism is causing it and what treatments are appropriate. This is particularly important in ensuring that the correct antibiotics are prescribed to treat bacterial infections which are appropriate for both the micro-organism and its possible resistance to some antibiotics.

Reasons for collecting microbiological specimens

Case study

Consider a woman admitted from a nursing home after falling and sustaining a hip fracture. She has a leg ulcer which is painful and producing green pus and needs to go to the operating theatre for her hip fracture to be attended to. She is also complaining of feeling hot and shivery and on recording her temperature you record it at 39°C.

In this case study there is more than one reason to obtain a microbiological sample. For example, the ulcer is showing signs and symptoms of infection so a swab needs to be obtained to see if it is infected. The patient has been admitted from a nursing home for surgery so needs a pre-operative MRSA screen. Her temperature is above 38°C which is an indication to obtain blood cultures (see later). All of these specimens, plus others, will be discussed in this chapter.

There are many reasons in healthcare why nurses may decide or be asked to obtain a microbiological specimen. Not all specimens collected are examined for the presence of micro-organisms – blood tests might be taken for a full blood count or liver function tests, for example – but this chapter focuses on specimens obtained for microbiological reasons. Specimens may be obtained:

- As a routine procedure on admission to some hospital wards – for example, some patients may be screened for MRSA or MSSA on admission to some wards, such as the intensive care unit.

- As a pre-operative check prior to some procedures.

- If there is an outbreak of infection on a ward or other settings such as a nursing home.

- If it is suspected that a patient has an infection based on signs and symptoms.

- To identify treatment options for an infection.

- To assess a patient after treatment – such as a repeat MRSA screen so see if the treatment has suppressed colonisation, though this has become less common due to long-term carriage in some patients.

- As part of sepsis screening.

Activity 6.1   *Reflection*

Consider specimens that you have obtained in previous practice placements. Why were these obtained and who decided that they were needed?

As this is based on your own experience, there is no answer provided for this activity.

You may have identified above quite a lot of specimens that you have obtained and a variety of reasons for doing so. You may also have found that you have obtained specimens without knowing the reason why. It is important to ensure that you know why you are obtaining a specimen – first, in case the patient asks, but primarily, you need to question if you should be undertaking any nursing activity if you do not understand why you are doing it. Having a rationale for your actions ensures that you are undertaking evidence-based nursing practice.

Types of microbiological specimen

As nurses we obtain a variety of samples from patients which we send to the laboratory for testing. These include swabs, blood tests and samples of other body fluids and excretions such as urine, faeces, sputum and joint fluids. If testing for bacteria, we request culture and sensitivity testing as this looks for both the bacteria and tests for antibiotic sensitivities for treatment purposes. For some organisms we need to ask for specific tests to be undertaken or these organisms may not be looked for in the laboratory. For example, if requesting a C&S (Culture and Sensitivity) on a faecal sample, *Clostridium difficile* may not be tested routinely so we need to ask for a *Clostridium difficile* toxin test. In some organisations, it is protocol to test all faecal samples for *Clostridium difficile* in patients over the age of two years, so you need to check this when on placement. Over time within your clinical placements you will become more familiar with the different tests which can be requested, including those outside the microbiology laboratory which are outside the remit of this chapter.

Swabs

Swabs may be taken from various sites on and in the body including wounds, the nose, throat, eye, rectum, penis and vagina. Some are also used in areas such as the groin and axillae, such as in screening for MRSA colonisation. When obtaining any type of swab, standard infection prevention and control precautions should be applied (see Chapter 8). You also need to consider, if testing for specific micro-organisms, that the patient may be suspected to have an infection for which isolation is required. If this is the case, it is usual practice to isolate until the laboratory confirms whether the patient has the infection or not.

Correctly obtaining swabs is important as, if undertaken incorrectly, results and therefore treatment can be affected.

Case study

The infection prevention and control nurse was called to a ward by the ward manager to see a patient with a crusty, weeping rash all over her face. Nurses had previously obtained a swab from the face, but this had come back from the laboratory with nothing abnormal found which was confusing the staff when the patient demonstrated clear signs of infection. On visiting the ward, the IPCN agreed that signs and symptoms of infection were present. However, on investigation it was discovered that the swab had been taken from one small area of the face. The site of swabbing therefore did not fully represent the widespread nature of the lesions. The IPCN obtained several swabs from the patient, including from each eye, forehead, each cheek and chin. These all returned from the laboratory positive for MRSA and treatment was prescribed for the patient.

As can be seen from the case study above, by not adequately obtaining the initial swab, treatment was delayed and symptoms continued. The *Marsden Manual* (Dougherty and Lister, 2015) provides evidence-based procedures for obtaining samples including swabs. You should be able to access a copy of this at your university, either in book form or online, and some NHS organisations use this manual as a basis for all their clinical procedures.

Wound swabs

Wound swabs are not usually obtained unless there are clinical signs and symptoms of infection. One of the reasons for this is that chronic wounds in particular can be heavily colonised with bacteria which are causing no infection – these would be identified from a swab but there would be no reason to treat the patient. We therefore, as previously mentioned, look for clinical signs and symptoms then obtain a specimen to confirm infection, what micro-organism is causing it and what the treatment options are. In general, when obtaining a wound swab, the swab should be rolled over the area of the wound. In some organisations it is usual practice to irrigate the wound with sterile saline prior to obtaining the swab to remove any surface debris such as dressing remnants. In large wounds, swabs may be obtained by moving the swab across the whole wound in a zig-zag motion to ensure that the whole surface of the wound is covered.

Wound swabs are usually obtained using a swab which contains a transport medium and needs to arrive at the laboratory within 24 hours. If the laboratory is closed, such as over a weekend or bank holiday, the swab should be stored in the refrigerator. Wound swabs are usually undertaken to look for bacteria, but may also be requested for fungal testing – if the latter, this needs to be indicated correctly on the request form. It is worth noting that in some organisations, wounds are included in admission screening so that if a patient is admitted with a wound present, it will be swabbed. Wound swabs are also taken as part of MRSA screening.

Throat swab

Obtaining a throat swab can activate the patient's gag reflex. It is therefore not advisable to obtain such a swab after a meal. A pen-torch may be required so that you can fully see the area to be swabbed, such as one tonsil or a yellow area of a tonsil. One swab should be used per tonsil so that if both tonsils need to be swabbed, two swabs are used. A tongue depressor may be needed to keep the tongue out of the way while the swab is rolled over the appropriate area. Throat swabs can be obtained to test for either bacteria or viruses and can be stored in the refrigerator out of hours.

Nasal swab

When the nose is being swabbed, one swab can be used for both nostrils. It is usual practice to moisten the swab first with sterile saline. When obtaining nasal swabs from babies, much smaller swabs are used and care needs to be taken with the delicate membranes inside the nose. Nasal swabs are obtained to test for bacteria.

High vaginal swab (HVS)

These are usually only obtained by qualified nurses or doctors, most often to investigate an abnormal discharge. A sterile **vaginal speculum** is needed so that the vaginal walls can be separated and the swab is used as high up in the vagina as possible. A strong light source is also needed during the process. An HVS is usually obtained to test for bacteria.

Rectal swab

These are commonly obtained in some organisations for CPE (Carbapenemase-Producing Enterobacteriaceae) or VRE (Vancomycin Resistant Enterococci) screening but can also be used to test for other bacteria, viruses and parasites. The swab is inserted into the rectum and rotated and the swab then returned immediately to the specimen container for transport to the laboratory.

MRSA screening

This generally includes a nasal swab as previously mentioned. If the perineum is swabbed, this involves rolling one swab over the area between the genitals and the anus. The swab is usually moistened first with sterile saline and the area may need to be cleaned prior to swabbing. In some organisations, a swab of the groin is obtained instead of the perineum – again the swab may be moistened with sterile saline and it should be rolled along the skin on the inner part of the thigh which is closest to the genitals. Whether or not to moisten the swab often depends on local policies so it is worth considering this in different placement areas.

Healthcare organisations routinely screen for MRSA for specific groups of patients on a risk assessment basis; for example, admissions to high-risk areas such as ICU, people admitted from nursing homes where colonisation rates are high, those who have previously had MRSA and those found to be MRSA positive in a site such as a wound, to check for colonisation in additional sites.

Activity 6.2   *Evidence-based practice and research*

Look at the MRSA screening policy in your current placement area. Who is routinely screened within the organisation? See if you can find out from a nurse on the ward why these particular people are screened.

There is no complete answer for this activity as the answer may be slightly different for each healthcare organisation, but some suggestions are made at the end of this chapter.

As a minimum, a swab is taken from the nose. In some organisations this may be the only swab taken during MRSA screening. In others it may also include areas such as the axillae, groins, open wounds, urine (particularly if a catheter is in situ) and the hairline.

Blood cultures

Blood cultures are taken to find out if a patient has a bacteraemia. It is common practice to obtain these cultures in patients who have a temperature above 38°C. There is a specific procedure to follow for obtaining blood cultures to ensure that the specimen obtained is not contaminated in any way – this could lead to a false positive result. Before obtaining the blood, the skin should be disinfected with a 2% chlorhexidine in 70% isopropyl alcohol swab and should be allowed to dry prior to needle insertion. The tops of the collection bottles should also be swabbed and allowed to dry. It is usual practice for blood cultures to be obtained in a set of two, with one bottle being tested for aerobic bacteria and the other anaerobic. Once these have been obtained they should be sent to the lab immediately. In some organisations, only specific staff can obtain blood cultures to minimise the contamination risk and specific training is usually provided. Some organisations will use a needle and syringe method and others a winged blood collection set method. It is worth familiarising yourself with both of these approaches and finding out in different placements who is permitted to obtain blood cultures. ANTT should be applied during the procedures (see Chapter 9). The *Marsden Manual* provides an evidence-based procedure for obtaining blood culture, though the technique may vary slightly between organisations.

Sputum specimens

Sputum specimens may be obtained for various microbiological tests to confirm chest infections and conditions such as pulmonary TB when patients have symptoms such as a productive cough, dyspnoea etc. How many sputum specimens are required, when they should be collected and what tests should be performed depends on what the doctor or nurse considers may be the source of a patient's symptoms and on set protocols such as in tuberculosis (TB) screening.

Sputum samples can be used to test for bacteria, fungi and parasites. Micro-organisms from the respiratory tract do not live for long periods of time outside the body and it is therefore important to transport the specimen to the laboratory soon after it being obtained. It is therefore beneficial, if you have provided a patient with a container in which to collect their sputum, that you advise them to let you know once they have provided their specimen. Alongside culture and sensitivity to test for bacteria, if there is a suspicion of tuberculosis, the sputum should be tested for acid fast bacilli (AAFB). In this latter case, three sputum specimens are required from three days in a row to increase the chance of the micro-organism being detected. If a patient is suspected to have pulmonary TB, until the laboratory confirms either way, both standard and transmission based precautions should be applied (Chapters 8 and 9).

Urine specimens

These are obtained to test for either bacteria, viruses or parasites.

Mid-stream urine (MSU)

This specimen involves the collection of the mid-point in a stream of urine. The patient is usually therefore instructed to discard the first part of the urine into the toilet or bedpan, then to pass the next portion into a sterile specimen container, with the remaining urine again discarded. Urine should arrive at the laboratory within 24 hours after being collected. Storage temperature depends on whether, for the test required, the urine has been obtained in a universal container (which can also be used for other body fluids) or a container with boric acid in it which acts as a preservative so that urine can be kept longer at room temperature. If the urine sample is to be tested for chlamydia, this needs to be stored in a refrigerator.

Early morning urine (EMU)

This is the same as an MSU but is the first urine passed that day. This is the best specimen for testing for mycobacteria (referred to in Chapter 3 in relation to tuberculosis) and for pregnancy testing. When testing for mycobacteria, urine should be obtained and tested from three consecutive days and be tested for acid fast bacilli.

Urine specimens from babies

It would be impractical to try to obtain an MSU from a baby. It is therefore usual for a collection bag to be secured over the genital area. Any urine collected is then transferred into a specimen container for transport to the laboratory.

Catheter specimen of urine (CSU)

When obtaining a urine specimen from a catheterised patient, this should only be done using the sampling port on the tubing using a sterile needle and syringe or, in many organisations, a sterile needleless connector syringe applying ANTT (Chapter 9). It is worth looking in your current placement what equipment is currently used for this procedure. Sterile containers are used in which to collect and transport the urine. DO NOT obtain the sample from the urine collection bag attached to the catheter. It is usually advised that 5–10 mL of urine be collected for testing.

Faecal samples

Faecal samples can be tested for bacteria such as salmonella species, viruses such as norovirus or parasites and are usually obtained when a patient has a history of diarrhoea. When there is a suspicion of *Clostridium difficile*, a toxin test is usually requested. When food poisoning is suspected it is common practice for three separate samples to be obtained from three separate bowel actions. Around 15 mL should be obtained if liquid faeces and it is acceptable to obtain the specimen from a bed pan which also contains urine.

Pus samples

These can be obtained from wounds or abscesses to be tested for bacteria. It usually involves the use of a sterile needle and syringe with which to extract the pus for testing.

Specimen labelling and request forms

Specimen request forms will look slightly different in different organisations.

Activity 6.3 　　　　　　　　　　*Evidence-based practice and research*

The next time that you are in a clinical placement, look at the specimen request forms on the ward or in the clinic. Familiarise yourself with what needs to be completed on the form.

No answer is provided for this activity as the answer will be different for each healthcare organisation.

Request forms will differ from one organisation to another but generally, labelling and transport requirements should be the same. The appropriate request form should be used (e.g. virology, bacteriology) depending on what you are wanting to test for. In some organisations, patient labels from notes can be used as labels on the specimen container: in other organisations, the labels on the containers need to be completed by hand with the patient name and hospital number, plus other information depending on the container. This should be checked with staff and policies in your placement areas. On request forms, the usual information required includes:

- The patient's full name
- Hospital ward or GP surgery
- NHS number
- Hospital number
- Tests required
- Date and time of collection of specimen
- Relevant patient information such as symptoms, any current antimicrobial treatment
- Source of specimen, e.g. eye swab.

The container with the specimen must be correctly sealed and labelled prior to placing it into the plastic pocket attached to the request form. If the specimen is leaking or the container is broken when it arrives at the laboratory, it will not be processed and another specimen will need to be obtained.

Danger of Infection/Infection Risk labels are usually applied to specimens from patients with high-risk (group 3 or 4) pathogens.

Activity 6.4   *Evidence-based practice and research*

Find out what pathogens are considered to be group 3 hazards for specimen labelling. You can find this information from the Advisory Committee on Dangerous Pathogens guidance (ACDP website address at the end of this chapter).

Some examples of these pathogens are found at the end of this chapter.

As you can see, there are quite a few organisms on this list. At this stage you might be questioning why we use these labels when we know a patient has one of these infections, but not on other patients when they might have the infection but we are not aware of it. This goes against the idea of standard precautions which are discussed in Chapter 8. Hazardous specimens are treated differently in the laboratory rather than all specimens being treated in this way. This is a health and safety requirement based on risk assessment and cost rather than a standard approach.

Transport of specimens

Wherever specimens are obtained from patients, once labelled and the request form has been completed, they need to be transported to the laboratory for testing. This may be from a ward or department in the same building as the laboratory or from another site, such as a clinic, a patient's home or another hospital. It is therefore important that the specimen is transported correctly to avoid spillages and delays and to comply with Health and Safety and Transport of Dangerous Goods legislation. When specimens are collected at ward level these are either collected by porters or transported to the laboratory by a member of ward staff. Some hospitals have a pneumatic delivery system, but these are usually not used for the transport of specimens from patients with group 3 or group 4 pathogens or suspected to have a TSE (transmissible spongiform encephalopathy, also known as prion disease). Where specimens are transported in cars or vans, they must be transported in a suitable transport box which is correctly labelled so that if there is an accident, specimens are contained within the box and people are aware of the contents. On some occasions, specimens are sent through the post. There are specific packaging arrangements for these depending on whether they are categorised as diagnostic or infectious samples.

Activity 6.5   *Critical thinking*

Farouk is admitted with a history of a productive cough, a raised temperature and night sweats. He has recently returned from a holiday in Pakistan with his family. On admission his temperature is 38.5°C and he is complaining of pain on passing urine.

What specimens would you obtain from this patient and what tests would you ask the laboratory to perform. Can you provide a rationale for your choices?

An example answer is provided at the end of this chapter.

Responding to results from the microbiology laboratory

Results are forwarded to the appropriate ward, department, clinic or GP surgery in various ways, including online, in paper form and via telephone, the latter when results are urgent and need to be acted on quickly. It is important as a healthcare practitioner/worker that if you are provided with laboratory results over the telephone that you document the date, time and results accurately and pass on the information as soon as possible to the appropriate staff member, be this a qualified nurse or doctor, so that appropriate action in terms of treatment and infection prevention and control precautions can be taken. When we obtain samples for culture and sensitivity, in addition to being provided with any positive findings of bacteria present, we are also provided with a list of antibiotics which the organism is sensitive to, that is, can be treated with. On a written form or on a computer screen this might appear as a list of antibiotics with either an S for sensitive or an R for resistant at the side of it. This enables the prescriber to make a choice about the best treatment for the infection, which can also be discussed with the consultant microbiologist.

Common terminology in microbiological testing

There are some terms which you will hear in nursing which relate to procedures within the microbiology laboratory. It is therefore valuable to have a basic understanding of what these mean, both for your own understanding and so that you can provide explanations to patients about what tests are being performed on the samples that they provide.

MC&S – this stands for 'microscopy, culture and sensitivity' and is what many samples obtained such as wound swabs, urine samples and so on are tested for. This test identifies what micro-organism(s) are present and identifies treatment options.

PCR – this stands for polymerase chain reaction. It is a process by which fragments of DNA are amplified so that detection of specific pathogens can be possible. It is a particularly important process in identifying genes related to antimicrobial resistance and is used in the detection of infections such as MRSA and HIV. It has in many ways vastly improved testing in terms of shortening the time taken to identify micro-organisms and is being used increasingly in the laboratory.

Genotyping – this is the process of determining differences in the genetic make-up by examining DNA and comparing to another organism or a reference sample. This can be useful in identifying the source of outbreaks of infection and therefore managing these outbreaks. For example, if several people have norovirus, it might be worth identifying whether these cases are linked – genotyping can be used in this way so that we can confirm an outbreak of infection rather than several unlinked cases.

Phage typing – this is a method used in the laboratory to detect single strains of bacteria within a species. It can be useful in situations such as when viruses that infect bacteria only infect one specific strain. It can therefore identify the source of outbreaks caused by specific strains of bacteria.

Serology – Serology testing is undertaken to detect antibodies to infection and can be used to detect changes in the number of antibodies produced, where the micro-organism causing the infection cannot be detected by MC&S and when the interaction between an antigen and antibody needs to be studied.

It is now time to test the knowledge that you have gained throughout this chapter with the usual multiple choice questions.

Activity 6.6 — Multiple choice and extended match questions

1. Which is the site most commonly swabbed in an MRSA screen?

    a) Groin
    b) Axilla
    c) Wound
    d) Nose
    e) Throat

2. Which of the following is a group 3 pathogen?

    a) *Clostridium difficile*
    b) MRSA
    c) *Pseudomonas aeruginosa*
    d) Hepatitis B
    e) *Candida albicans*

3. For which of the following organisms would a rectal swab be obtained?

    a) CPE
    b) MRSA

c) *Clostridium difficile*

d) *Candida albicans*

e) Malaria

For each of the questions below, one of the following answers is correct. The same answer may be correct for more than one question.

A   Wound swab

B   Nose swab

C   MSU

D   Sputum specimen

E   Rectal swab

F   Faeces for bacteriology

Which of the samples above would be obtained in the following situations:

1. A 78-year-old lady admitted from a nursing home after a fall.
2. A patient complaining of pain on passing urine, a high temperature and passing urine more frequently than usual.
3. A patient with a history of diarrhoea after recently returning from abroad.
4. A patient with a productive cough.
5. A patient on a ward where other patients have been found to have CPE.

Answers at the end of the chapter.

In addition to the usual multiple choice type question you have now also been exposed to an EMQ (extended match question), which is commonly used in multiple choice examination papers.

Chapter summary

In this chapter we have briefly considered some of the specimens which we, as nurses, might obtain from patients for microbiological testing and how these should be labelled and transported. We have also considered some of the tests which might be performed on these tests by the laboratory. You should now be more aware of the link between the symptoms and signs of infection that we have previously discussed, the micro-organisms which cause infection, and how we might test for these in order to better manage and treat our patients.

Activities: Brief outline answers

Activity 6.2: Evidence-based practice and research (page 97)

Some examples of people who may be screened for MRSA in different hospitals include those admitted from other countries (as resistance patterns may be different), those transferred from other hospitals (as strains may be different in different areas of the country), those admitted from long-term care facilities (as colonisation rates can be high), those previously found to have MRSA (as colonisation might have recurred) and those admitted to high-risk areas such as ICU/ITU, renal units, vascular surgery etc. (as these patients are at higher risk of serious infections if MRSA spreads) – this list will differ between organisations.

Activity 6.4: Evidence-based practice and research (page 100)

Some examples of group 3 pathogens include *E. coli* 0157, *Mycobacterium tuberculosis, Salmonella paratyphi, Yersinia pestis, Blastomyces dermatitidis, Histoplasma capsulatum, Plasmodium falciparum,* CJD, FFI, GSS, SARS, hepatitis C, hepatitis B, hepatitis E.

Activity 6.5: Critical thinking (page 101)

Farouk is admitted with a history of a productive cough, a raised temperature and night sweats. He has recently returned from a holiday in Pakistan with his family. On admission his temperature is 38.5°C and he is complaining of pain on passing urine.

What specimens would you obtain from this patient and what tests would you ask the laboratory to perform. Can you provide a rationale for your choices?

You might have suggested obtaining blood cultures due to his temperature being above 38°C, a urine specimen for C&S due to pain on passing urine, and sputum specimens to test for both routine culture and AAFB (acid fast bacilli) to test for *Mycobacterium tuberculosis* due to returning from an area of prevalence.

Activity 6.6 Multiple choice/extended match questions (pages 102–3)

1. Which is the site most commonly swabbed in an MRSA screen?

    d) Nose

2. Which of the following is a group 3 pathogen?

    d) Hepatitis B

3. For which of the following organisms would a rectal swab be obtained?

    a) CPE

Which of the samples listed would be obtained in the following situations:

1. A 78-year-old lady admitted from a nursing home after a fall: B (for MRSA screening)

2. A patient complaining of pain on passing urine, a high temperature and passing urine more frequently than usual: C

3. A patient with a history of diarrhoea after recently returning from abroad: F

4. A patient with a productive cough: D

5. A patient on a ward where other patients have been found to have CPE: E

Further reading

Dougherty, L and Lister, S (2015) *The Royal Marsden Manual of Clinical Nursing Procedures,* 9th edition. Chichester: John Wiley.

This book has chapters relating to microbiological specimens which are easy to understand.

Garner, D (2014) *Microbiology Nuts and Bolts: Key Concepts of Microbiology and Infection,* 2nd edition. Amazon: Createspace.

This manual provides evidence-based procedures for obtaining a variety of microbiological specimens. Many local procedures and guidelines are based on this manual.

Murray, PR (ed.) (2007) *Manual of Clinical Microbiology,* 9th edition. Washington DC: ASM Press.

This book provides in-depth information about laboratory techniques for those students with a specific interest.

Useful website

www.gov.uk/government/groups/advisory-committee-on-dangerous-pathogens

This is the website for the Advisory Committee on Dangerous Pathogens which publishes some of the guidance on laboratory specimens.

Chapter 7
Roles and responsibilities in infection prevention and control

Chapter aims

After reading this chapter, you will be able to:

- Describe the roles of the different members of the infection prevention and control team.
- Understand the role of the link nurse/link practitioner.
- Be aware of some of the national documents available which support infection prevention and control in clinical practice.

Throughout this book so far we have focused primarily on the microbiology related aspects of nursing. Before we look at infection prevention and control (IPC) precautions which are applied to patients in healthcare settings, this chapter will introduce you to staff who can be a source of advice, information and support to you in relation to infection while you are in your clinical placements. The chapter will begin by discussing the roles and responsibilities of the infection prevention and control team before discussing specific roles within the team. It will then consider the link practitioner role before discussing some of the important recent documents in the UK which have an impact on infection prevention and control and which it will be useful for you to be aware of, both as a student and when you register as a practitioner at the end of your course.

Scenario

Jane is a student nurse in her second ward placement. On her third week, the ward is visited by inspectors from the Care Quality Commission. As a student, Jane thinks that these inspectors are not there to speak to her, but instead will focus on what the qualified staff and patients have to say. However, one of the inspectors smiles at her and asks her, informally, about the staff available within the organisation in which she is placed who can provide her with advice about infection prevention and control when she is not sure what to do as a first year student. She is also asked if there are any documents that she can read to learn more about what is recommended in the UK in terms of infection prevention and control practice to support her learning and practices. As Jane has been caring for a patient in isolation with an infection, she is able to tell the inspector about some of the different dedicated staff within the organisation who play a role in infection prevention in terms of support and advice and about the national evidence-based guidelines for infection prevention in the hospital setting.

Consider the above scenario. In this position, would you be able to respond to the inspector? You may consider that responding to such questions is not particularly important, but knowing about sources of support on the wards and what national guidelines are available is valuable for you both as a student and when you register as a practitioner and for other professions outside of nursing. This is also information which is important in supporting the care of patients so that we are aware of who both we and they can contact for advice and support and that there are systems of support in place.

The infection prevention and control team (IPCT)

Each NHS organisation has a team of people responsible for IPC. This team has a variety of roles within the organisation, but work together to support its IPC infrastructure and services, reporting to the Trust Board and the chief executive. They are often all members of the IPC committee which meets on a regular basis and produces the organisation's annual programme for IPC activity and annual report to provide information to the Board about where the organisation is in relation to its programme, what healthcare-associated infections have been an issue within the previous year and what actions need to be taken to improve things in relation to IPC.

It is a requirement under the Code of Practice which is part of the Health and Social Care Act 2008 (DH, 2015) that healthcare organisations either have or have access to an appropriate mix of expertise in relation to IPC – the IPCT fulfils this requirement. As can be seen here, it is not only NHS organisations which need to have access to such expertise. Non-NHS organisations may have their own IPCT or may contract for the use of a local NHS team, in particular in relation to microbiology advice. The IPCT in the NHS includes people such as the IPC doctor, consultant microbiologist (these two may be the same person) and IPC nurse/practitioner (IPCN/P).

The infection prevention and control doctor (IPCD)

Within NHS organisations, someone is designated as the infection control doctor. This might be the consultant microbiologist, public health doctor or infectious diseases consultant. Whoever this person may be, they are seen as the lead for the IPCT. The role of IPCD is not full time but this person often chairs the infection prevention and control committee and liaises closely with the infection prevention and control nurse.

The infection prevention and control nurse/practitioner (IPCN/P)

This person may often be the only full-time member of the IPCT. In many organisations there is now a team of nurses within the IPCT; in smaller organisations, such as Mental Health or Care Trusts there may only be one. The IPC nurse/practitioner fulfils a variety of roles including the provision of IPC related advice to all staff within the organisation, clinical audit, risk management, surveillance, staff education, outbreak management and policy and guideline development (Quattrin et al., 2004; Weston, 2013). The IPCP is usually the first point of contact for IPC advice within organisations and is the most visible clinical person within the IPCT. IPCPs work differently within organisations. In some NHS Trusts, IPCPs are allocated to specific divisions so that staff on specific wards have a named member of the IPCT to contact. For example, one IPCP may cover surgery, another medicine, another critical care settings and so on. In other organisations, nurses may take on specific roles so that one IPCN undertakes all the audit, another all the surveillance and so on. Within each of your clinical placements it is worth identifying your point of contact for IPC advice within that area. It has been identified that the presence of an IPCN/P can both improve practice and reduce rates of infection (Venberghe et al., 2002; Ward, 2012).

The first infection prevention and control nurse was employed in the UK in 1959.

Scenario

Jack is a mental health nurse working on an acute ward. One of his patients is admitted after a suicide attempt and this patient has a history of self-harm. There are multiple lacerations on the patient's body, one of which is showing signs of infection. A swab is obtained and the patient is found to have MRSA.

Jack has not had any experience with MRSA for a long time as it is not a common infection on the ward where he works. He is therefore unsure what he should do next. However, he has a good relationship with the infection prevention and control practitioner who covers his ward area and contacts them for advice. The IPCP is able to provide him with information about further screening required to check for colonisation, standard precautions required, whether he needs to be isolated in a side room and treatment options. The IPCP also offers to come to the ward to speak to the patient and his relatives so that they can ask any questions they have about MRSA.

As can be seen from this scenario, one of the important roles of the IPCP is in providing advice and information, to staff, patients and their relatives. They are a vital point of contact for all staff and it is therefore important to be aware of who the IPCN is for your placement area and how this person can be contacted.

The consultant microbiologist

This member of staff will provide advice related to the medical aspects of patient management. This might include advice about the prescribing of antibiotics, translating laboratory reports, advising doctors on treatment and so on and medically reviewing patients with infections. This consultant may or may not also be the infection control doctor, but will generally be a member of the IPCT and sit on the IPC committee.

Outside of the NHS acute hospital Trust setting, the IPC team may function differently. Previously there was the Health Protection Agency which had a nurse and doctor who worked locally, taking responsibility for IPC matters outside the NHS such as in nursing and residential homes. Primary Care Trusts also often employed their own IPC practitioner to cover services such as community nursing, podiatry and dentistry. However, primary and community care provision has changed with the creation of Clinical Commissioning Groups. Community IPC practitioners may now be employed by a variety of organisations such as the CCGs themselves, local councils and acute Trusts who provide IPC services to primary care. This can cause confusion about who to contact for staff working in primary care so good communication within and between services is important to ensure that all staff know who their first point of contact is for IPC. In some areas, health protection or public health nurses may provide IPC input alongside other health protection related responsibilities. Mental Health and Care Trusts function very much like acute Trusts in most cases in relation to IPC provision, employing their own IPC practitioners.

The director of infection prevention and control

This role is required under the Health and Social Care Act 2008 (Department of Health, 2015) and should be in place in all registered NHS care providers. The person undertaking this role is generally not in a full-time or unique role, but it is undertaken alongside another role. However, time should be allocated for the person to fulfil the requirements of this role. The DIPC needs to be an effective leader who is highly visible, senior and authoritative. The DIPC in particular provides assurance to the Trust Board that systems are in place within the organisation to ensure safe and effective healthcare, though they do not need to be a member of the Trust Board. They should, however, report directly to the chief executive.

Considering recent changes within the NHS, the role of the DIPC will differ when working for either commissioning (such as Clinical Commissioning Groups) or provider (such as an NHS hospital) organisations. Provider organisations are expected to have their own DIPC to provide information and assurance to the board. In commissioning organisations, the role will involve providing advice on service specifications and performance indicators related to provider contracts. While there is no single model for how the role of the DIPC is provided within each organisation, the commitment to patient safety and quality care should be paramount. The DIPC role can be undertaken by microbiologists, directors of public health, infection prevention and control practitioners, directors of nursing, medical directors and so on – each organisation will be different.

Activity 7.1   *Evidence-based practice and research*

Find out in your current placement organisation who the DIPC is. What other job role does this person undertake? Do the staff where you are working know who the DIPC is?

There is no answer provided for this activity as it will be dependent on your placement organisation.

You may have found that people working within the organisation did not know that this person was the DIPC. The DIPC should ideally be the public face of infection prevention and control within an organisation and should therefore be known to everyone working within in.

The infection prevention and control link nurse/practitioner (IPCLN/P)

Link nurses/practitioners are used frequently in healthcare settings to support many areas of specialist practice in the UK, including diabetes, pain management and tissue viability. The link nurse role was introduced into infection prevention in 1988 by Rozila Horton; these are practising nurses who have an interest in a specific area of nursing and act as a formal link to the specialist team for that area within the organisation. The role is used in different ways within organisations, with activities and responsibility varying. Titles can be different, requirements to undertake the role can vary and how effective the role is can be dependent on many issues such as the person undertaking the role, how they are perceived by their colleagues and how well they are supported by the IPCT. Not all link staff are nurses. For example, in departments where nurses are not employed, such as podiatry, the link person might be referred to as a link practitioner. In a basic sense, the role of the link person is to act as a bridge between the IPCT and clinical staff, sharing knowledge and good practice, and sometimes being involved in clinical audits, surveillance and the education of staff in their work area. Four key themes for the role have been identified by the RCN (2012a): acting as a role model for IPC; enabling others to learn and develop their IPC practice; communication and networking around IPC practice; and supporting others in local audit and surveillance, though the last theme is considered optional due to the differing nature of healthcare organisations. Though there is a lack of evidence about the efficacy of link staff, some studies have highlighted benefits to having link systems in place in infection prevention and control (Miyachi et al., 2007; Seto et al., 2013; Lloyd Smith et al., 2014).

Activity 7.2 *Reflection*

Think of the placements that you have experienced so far. Was there a link nurse/practitioner in your placements? If so, what did this nurse/practitioner do and how was he or she perceived by the other staff members?

There is no answer for this activity as this will be dependent on placement experience.

In some areas you may be able to clearly identify the person in this role and in others not. You may have also been to practice areas which have no designated IPCLN – this is not a mandatory role and some organisations have taken the decision not to utilise it due to a lack of efficacy in their areas. However, in some areas the use of link nurses can mean that problems are identified and addressed more quickly.

Case study

In one town in the North of England there is a link nurse system in the local nursing homes (including adult, mental health and learning disability homes). Some of the homes have an ICPLN/P and some do not. These practitioners have regular meetings with the community IPCP and receive a monthly newsletter. One link nurse informs the IPCP that they have an outbreak of diarrhoea and vomiting in Ashwood Court (pseudonym), the adult and dementia care nursing home where she works, which the nurse thinks may be caused by norovirus infection. The IPCP visits the home to meet with the link nurse and offer advice about staff movement, isolation of affected residents, cleaning procedures and staff sickness. The link practitioner works with the IPCP and is in contact with her on a daily basis. The outbreak is over a week later. Two weeks after this, another home which does not have a link practitioner contacts the IPCP to say that they have an outbreak of diarrhoea and vomiting which has been ongoing for several weeks, has affected most of the residents and has resulted in seven staff being affected and off sick. As there is no link practitioner, there was no immediate action by the home once an outbreak had been recognised and advice was not sought until the outbreak was widespread affecting both residents and staff.

As can be seen from the above case study, having a link practitioner in place can lead to a quicker resolution to problematic issues such as outbreaks of infection. Having staff with a greater level of knowledge in these areas who have a link and direct relationship with the local IPCP can be of benefit to both patients and staff in such situations.

The infection prevention and control committee

As previously mentioned, NHS organisations generally have an infection prevention and control committee (IPCC) which meets on a regular basis and reports to the Trust Board. Its members vary between organisations but will include the members of the IPC team and other people such as the Chief Nurse, Medical Director, Occupational Health Lead, Health and Safety and Clinical Governance representatives and other people in senior roles within the organisation. The role of the IPCC is multi-faceted and will include planning, monitoring, evaluating, updating and educating in relation to IPC. It sets general IPC policy and provides input into specific IPC issues. Simply stated, its function is to prevent and control healthcare-associated infections. That is accomplished in a variety of ways, some of which include: surveillance of infections, product evaluation, investigation of infection outbreaks and development of IPC procedures.

National documents

Over the past 20 years, multiple documents have been published by organisations such as the Department of Health, NICE, Health Protection Scotland, Public Health Wales, NHS Scotland and Public Health England in relation to infection prevention and control. This chapter does not aim to talk about all of these, but instead will focus on the most recent and important publications which it would be beneficial for you to have some knowledge and understanding of. These include the epic3 guidelines, NICE IPC guidelines for primary care and the Health and Social Care Act 2008: Code of Practice on the prevention and control of infections and related guidance.

epic3 (Loveday et al., 2014)

This document provides the most recent evidence-based infection prevention and control guidelines for use in hospital settings. The document provides both recommendations, and the evidence base for each of these so that we can see what research and expert support is available for each action that we take in IPC. It covers standard principles, environmental hygiene, hand hygiene, the use of personal protective equipment, sharps management, asepsis and guidelines on IPC in short-term urinary catheterisation and the use of intravenous access devices. Each recommendation within the guidelines is allocated a category from A to D depending on the type of evidence which supports it. This is the third version of hospital-based guidelines from epic and provides the basis for policies and guidelines within healthcare settings which should ideally refer to these guidelines as part of their evidence base. The epic guidelines are reviewed regularly so you need to ensure that you access the most up-to-date guidelines.

NICE guidelines: Prevention and control of healthcare-associated infections in primary and community care (NICE, 2012)

NICE has been responsible for the national evidence-based guidelines for IPC in primary and community care settings. Many of the recommendations are similar to those in the epic3 guidelines as most of the main principles are the same, but there are some differences to ensure that recommendations are relevant to settings outside of acute hospitals. To be consistent with epic, the NICE guidelines also cover standard principles, hand decontamination, urinary catheterisation (including intermittent self-catheterisation) and vascular access devices. NICE also identifies key priorities for implementation in terms of the recommendations within the guidelines and makes a differentiation between the words 'must' and 'should' within the guidance. 'Must' generally relates to recommendations which have legal ramifications if not met. There is a great emphasis within the document on the education of both healthcare workers and patients (and their carers) to ensure that everyone involved in care in community settings has knowledge about IPC.

The first NICE guidelines for IPC were produced in 2003, but they were reviewed due to changes within NHS provision and the fact that increasingly complex care is being carried out in primary and community care settings. There is also a stated assumption within the guidelines that all providers of healthcare in both primary and community care settings are fully compliant with the Code of Practice discussed below. NICE guidelines are reviewed so you need to ensure that you access the most up-to-date documents on their website: **www.nice.org.uk**.

The Health and Social Care Act 2008: Code of Practice for the prevention and control of infections and related guidance (Department of Health, 2015)

This document was produced

> [t]o help providers of healthcare, including primary dental care, primary medical care, adult social care, and independent sector ambulance providers, plan and implement how they prevent and control infections. It includes criteria for CQC to take into account when assessing compliance with the registration requirement on cleanliness and infection control.

The Code also highlights the following:

> The law states that the Code must be taken into account by the CQC when it makes decisions about registration against the cleanliness and infection control requirement. The regulations also say that providers must have regard to the Code when deciding how they will comply with registration requirements. So, by following the Code, registered providers will be able to show that they meet the requirement set out in the regulations. However, the Code is not mandatory so registered providers do not by law have to comply with the Code. A registered provider may be able to demonstrate that it meets the regulations in a different way (equivalent or better) from that described in this document. The Code aims to exemplify what providers need to do in order to comply with the regulations.

Therefore, while it is not a legal requirement for healthcare providers to comply with the Code, doing so will ensure that they meet their registration standards. It is therefore within the interests of these organisations to be compliant with the Code.

The Code includes 10 compliance criteria which registered providers need to demonstrate that they meet. These are related to issues such as the provision of a clean environment, provision of advice to patients and visitors, adherence to IPC policies, management of occupational health needs and the provision of isolation facilities.

Activity 7.3   *Evidence-based practice and research*

Go online and find a copy of the above Code of Practice. What does the document say about the following issues:

- Risk assessment in relation to compliance with criterion 1?
- What policies on the environment should be addressed in criterion 2?
- What policies should be available under criterion 9?

There is no model answer to this question as the answers will be the result of your own research.

As can be seen, the Code covers a lot of relevant aspects. It is therefore worth considering whether your placements meet the requirements of the Code.

It is now time to review what you have learned within this chapter.

Activity 7.4   *Multiple choice questions*

1. Who is usually considered to be the lead for the infection prevention and control team?

    a) The infection prevention and control nurse
    b) The infection prevention and control link nurse
    c) The ward manager
    d) The infection prevention and control doctor
    e) The chief executive

2. For which setting are the epic3 guidelines meant?

    a) GP surgeries
    b) Hospitals
    c) Community nursing
    d) The private sector
    e) The operating theatre

---

3. In the NICE guidelines, what does the word 'must' relate to?

    a) Key priorities for implementation
    b) What NICE would recommend that staff do
    c) Recommendations which relate to patient education
    d) Recommendations which have legal ramifications if not met
    e) Recommendations which relate to catheter care

4. How many compliance criteria are there in the Code of Practice related to the Health and Social Care Act?

    a) 5
    b) 10
    c) 15
    d) 20
    e) 25

Chapter summary

In this chapter we have considered the roles of the main people involved in IPC at a higher level within NHS organisations and have identified some of the key documents in relation to IPC. These provide you with a basis on which to build throughout your career in identifying sources of help, support, advice and information related to infection prevention and control.

Activities: Brief outline answers

Activity 7.4: MCQs (pages 114–15)

1. Who is usually considered to be the lead for the infection prevention and control team?

    d) The infection prevention and control doctor

2. For which setting are the epic3 guidelines meant?

    b) Hospitals

3. In the NICE guidelines, what does the word 'must' relate to?

    d) Recommendations which have legal ramifications if not met

4. How many compliance criteria are there in the Code of Practice related to the Health and Social Care Act?

    b) 10

Further reading

Royal College of Nursing (2012) *The role of the link nurse in infection prevention and control (IPC): developing a link nurse framework.* London: RCN.

This document provides guidance for what should be required of link nurses in IPC, including competencies.

Useful websites

www.his.org.uk/files/3113/8693/4808/epic3_National_Evidence-Based_Guidelines_for_Preventing_HCAI_in_NHSE.pdf

Hospital Infection Society direct link to the epic3 guidelines.

www.nice.org.uk/guidance/cg139/resources/guidance-infection-pdf

NICE direct link to the NICE guidelines on IPC in primary and community care.

www.gov.uk/government/publications/the-health-and-social-care-act-2008-code-of-practice-on-the-prevention-and-control-of-infections-and-related-guidance

Direct link to the Code of Practice from the Health and Social Care Act 2008 Code of Practice.

Chapter 8
Standard infection prevention and control precautions

continued . . . •••

- Applies knowledge of an 'exposure prone procedure' and takes appropriate precautions and action (Progression point 2).
- Takes personal responsibility, when a student knowingly has a blood-borne virus, to consult occupational health before carrying out exposure prone procedures (Progression point 2).
- Adheres to infection prevention and control policies and procedures at all times and ensures that colleagues work according to good practice guidelines (Progression point 3).
- Manages overall environment to minimise risk (Progression point 3).

Chapter aims

After reading this chapter, you will be able to:

- Identify the standard precautions which should be applied to all patients.
- Demonstrate the correct way to decontaminate hands, using both soap and alcohol hand rub.
- Distinguish between the different types of personal protective equipment and when they should be used.
- Identify the categories of risk for decontamination and suggest appropriate decontamination approaches for items within each of these categories.
- Identify the steps to safely manage sharps and to deal effectively with a sharps injury.
- Discuss some of the ways in which body fluid spillages may be managed.

In previous chapters we have considered the micro-organisms which cause infections in humans. It is now time to look at ways in which we, as nurses, can prevent infection and cross-infection in different healthcare settings. In this chapter we will first look at the background to standard precautions and how they may be classified. In turn we will then look at hand hygiene, the use of personal protective equipment, sharps management, decontamination and blood and body fluid spillage management. Throughout the chapter there are activities and scenarios to enable you to apply your knowledge to practice situations and to test what you have learned throughout the chapter.

Scenario

Thomas is a 48-year-old patient with a history of self-harm. He is visited by various members of the multi-disciplinary team to meet his physical, psychological and social needs in his own home. He has recently been discharged from hospital following an admission for a self-harming episode in which a deep laceration was caused to his left arm which has been sutured closed. He is visited three times weekly by the community psychiatric nurse and twice weekly by the district nurse to dress his wound and eventually to remove the sutures. Considering what has been learned from previous chapters, Thomas is at risk of infection because of his mental health and because he has a wound. He is also not attending very well to his nutritional needs. In the few days since his discharge from hospital he has removed his sutures on one occasion which required an A&E visit for re-suturing. During this episode, his living room was contaminated with blood from his wound. As a nurse visiting his home, you need to ensure that neither Thomas nor yourself are put at risk of infection. You can do this by applying the standard precautions that we are going to discuss in this chapter.

As can be seen from this scenario, consideration of infection risks and the application of precautions which reduce these risks is relevant in settings outside of acute hospitals. As nurses we therefore need to be able to apply infection prevention and control (IPC) principles in a variety of settings, some of which are not necessarily considered to be clinical, including a patient's own home.

Standard IPC precautions

Depending on where in the UK you live, these may be referred to as either standard precautions or standard infection prevention and control precautions, but both terms refer to the same thing. IPC precautions have developed over time, particularly in response to the discovery of the HIV virus. Universal precautions were introduced in the mid-1980s as a response to this. The basic view was that all patients and their body fluids should be treated as a source of infection, whether known to have an infection or not, as we cannot tell, by looking at someone, whether or not they are HIV positive. However, this applies to other blood-borne viruses and micro-organisms. Risks are also associated with open wounds and mucous membranes. We now have what is referred to as standard (IPC) precautions which apply to all patients, their body fluids, mucous membranes and open wounds. These precautions should be applied to everyone, rather than selectively on patients who we know have an infection. Think back to earlier chapters of different types of micro-organism and normal flora – we do not know what micro-organisms we personally carry on or inside our bodies and neither do our patients. This best approach therefore assumes that everyone could pose a significant risk.

Standard IPC precautions include hand decontamination, the use of personal protective equipment, sharps management, decontamination and body fluid spillage management, all of which will be covered in this chapter.

Transmission based precautions (TBP)

Transmission based precautions are an additional set of measures that should be implemented when patients/clients are either suspected or known to be infected with a specific infectious agent. These precautions are categorised according to the route of transmission of the infectious agent such as droplet, contact and/or airborne. Transmission based precautions are needed because the transmission of some infectious agents is not prevented by the application of standard IPC precautions alone, for example *Mycobacterium tuberculosis*. While standard precautions should be applied to all patients, transmission based precautions are the extra precautions which are applied in addition to the basic standard precautions in specific infections.

According to Health Protection Scotland (HPS, 2015), transmission based precautions are required in all health and social care settings when a patient or client is known or suspected to be infected or colonised with an infectious agent that can be spread by the droplet, contact and/or airborne routes, such as MRSA or *Clostridium difficile* as these may spread and cause harm to others, such as patients or staff, while care is being delivered to them. TBP are categorised as contact, droplet or airborne precautions.

- *Contact precautions*: Used to prevent and control infections that spread via direct contact with the patient or indirectly from the patient's immediate care environment (including care equipment). This might include infections such as *Clostridium difficile*, salmonella and MRSA. In these cases, additional precautions are applied when having direct physical contact with these patients such as the wearing of gloves and aprons (discussed later) which is additional to the use of such items in the standard approach.

- *Droplet precautions*: Used to prevent and control infections spread over short distances (at least 3 feet (1 metre)) via droplets from the respiratory tract of one individual directly onto a mucosal surface or conjunctivae of another individual. This includes infections such as whooping cough, mumps, norovirus, parvovirus B19, rotavirus and influenza virus. Additional precautions would include isolation of the patient.

- *Airborne precautions*: Used to prevent and control infections spread without necessarily having close patient contact via aerosols from the respiratory tract of one individual directly onto a mucosal surface or conjunctivae of another individual. This would include infections such as pulmonary tuberculosis, measles and chicken pox. Additional precautions would include isolation.

The HPS national IPC manual contains information about which infectious agents might require transmission based precautions such as isolation in a single room (see website information at the end of this chapter), cohorting, the use of masks etc. Further information on isolation can be found in Chapter 9. These precautions need to be considered, however, based on the setting in which the patient is being cared for as risk assessment needs to be undertaken in settings such as nursing homes, the patient's own home and in more acute areas such as the intensive care unit. Information on isolation and cohorting can be found in the next chapter. There can be problems with staff understanding when TBPs should be applied (Russell et al., 2014) and it is therefore something which you need to gain experience of in practice.

Hand hygiene/decontamination

Hand hygiene/decontamination (including both hand washing and the use of alcohol hand rub) is the most important intervention in the control of cross-infection due to the fact that most cross-infection in healthcare settings is caused by the transfer of micro-organisms on staff hands. Ignaz Semmelweiss is credited with the discovery of the value of hand hygiene in the prevention of cross-infection in 1847 in the obstetrics setting.

There are many occasions when hand hygiene should be undertaken as a nurse. The World Health Organization identified the five moments for hand hygiene which are generally specific to the acute setting.

Activity 8.1 *Evidence-based practice and research*

Go online to the WHO website and find the WHO's five moments for hand hygiene. What are these five moments?

Answers can be found at the end of the chapter.

Different activities can be included in each of these five moments. The occasions when hands should be decontaminated are vast and are therefore not listed here. However, the main principles of the WHO moments should be considered – if the occasion fits into one of these five moments, then hands should be decontaminated in the acute setting. There are clearly multiple additional occasions when hands should be decontaminated including after glove removal, after going to the toilet and before food preparation.

Prior to hand decontamination

In order to promote effective hand hygiene, healthcare organisations promote what they refer to as a 'bare below the elbows' policy. This term was translated from initial Department of Health guidance on uniforms, though the term never appeared in the guidelines. It is therefore recommended that staff undertaking clinical/patient care activities have nothing in terms of clothing or jewellery below their elbows. For those staff wearing their own clothes who undertake clinical procedures, this might mean rolling up sleeves. For all staff this also means no jewellery on the wrists or hands when undertaking clinical procedures or decontaminating hands, plus wearing no nail polish and having short nails. There are various reasons for these requirements:

- Most microbes on the hands are found on and around the fingernails. This means that the longer the nails, the bigger the potential for microbes on the hands. Fingernails should therefore be kept short by clinical staff.

- False nails increase the surface area for microbes, inhibit a proper hand hygiene technique due to fear of them falling off and can harbour liquid between the false and real nail which encourages bacterial and fungal growth (Gordin et al., 2007).

- Wrist watches can become contaminated and inhibit the decontamination of the wrists during hand hygiene.

- Stoned rings can become contaminated with micro-organisms, are difficult to clean and can cause tears in gloves (Ward, 2007).
- Nail polish flakes off, causing ridges on the nails which can harbour micro-organisms.

(Fagernes and Linges, 2011)

Some organisations allow a plain wedding band, but this should be removed or moved up during hand hygiene procedures. You also need to ensure that cuts and abrasions on your hands are covered by a waterproof dressing to avoid infection.

How hands should be decontaminated

There are different approaches to hand decontamination, with different products being used depending on what the aim is. Hand hygiene is generally divided into routine and surgical – these two types require different products and different lengths of time plus they aim to remove different types of flora from the hands.

Routine hand hygiene

This is the type of hand hygiene performed in most care situations involving the nurse with the aim of removing transient micro-organisms, that is, those which are temporary on the hands, are easily transferred from one person to another and which cause most of the cross-infection in healthcare settings. As these micro-organisms are easily transferred to other people and inanimate objects, they are also relatively easy to remove from the hands using the correct technique. The technique is the same for routine hand hygiene whether liquid soap or alcohol hand rub is being used. NICE (2012) and epic3 (Loveday et al., 2014) both advocate the use of alcohol hand rub for routine hand decontamination unless:

- Hands are visibly soiled or dirty (in this case the alcohol may be inactivated by the matter on the hands).
- Caring for a patient with a suspected or known gastro-intestinal infection such as norovirus, a spore-forming organism such as *Clostridium difficile* (as alcohol does not destroy spores) or CPE (NICE, 2012; Loveday et al., 2014; Weston, 2013), though there are other indications for the use of soap and water outside of the clinical sphere such as after going to the toilet.

In the above situations, hands should be washed using a liquid soap – it does not need to contain an antiseptic. Bar soap should not be used in clinical settings as it quickly becomes contaminated. When using liquid soap, hands should be washed as follows:

- Wet hands under running water.
- Apply soap (usually only one shot is needed from the dispenser).
- Wash all areas of the hands.
- Rinse the soap off fully.
- Completely dry the hands.

Undertaking the procedure in this way reduces the risk of sore dry skin on the hands, thereby reducing the risk of increased bacterial counts on hands associated with this dry skin. In settings where the above situations occur but there is no appropriate source of running water, it is acceptable to use hand wipes followed by alcohol hand rub.

In terms of decontaminating all areas of the hands, this also applies when using alcohol hand rub for routine hand hygiene. There is a specific technique for this developed by Ayliffe et al. in 1978 and since extended. This technique was developed after acknowledgement that when staff in healthcare undertook hand hygiene there were certain areas that they missed during the procedure, in particular the thumbs, tips of the fingers, between the fingers and thumbs and the wrists. This technique ensures that all areas of the hands are decontaminated. The steps within the procedure can be undertaken in any order, but the wrists must be decontaminated last.

Activity 8.2   *Reflection*

In your university or your placement area, look to see if there is a piece of equipment called a hand inspection cabinet/light box. If you have not used one of these before, see if you can now use it – it will identify to you which areas of your hands you miss when you wash your hands. In some areas of practice you may also find other computer-based programmes which you can try relating to hand hygiene.

Which areas did you miss?

There is no answer for this activity as it involves you reflecting on what you have done.

As you may have identified from the activity above, we miss areas when we wash our hands. Using specific steps will ensure that all areas of the hands are decontaminated. The steps within hand decontamination, after ensuring that you are bare below the elbows are as follows:

- Rub your hands together palm to palm.

- Rub your right palm over the back of your left hand then your left palm over the back of your right hand.

- Rub your palms together with your fingers interlaced.

- Rub the backs of your fingers on your opposing palms with fingers interlocked.

- Rub each thumb in the opposite palm.

- Rub in a rotational action with the clasped fingers of one hand in the palm of the opposite hand then vice versa.

- Rub each wrist with the opposite hand.

This technique should take between 10 and 15 seconds when using soap and water and is complete once the hand rub is dried when using alcohol hand rub.

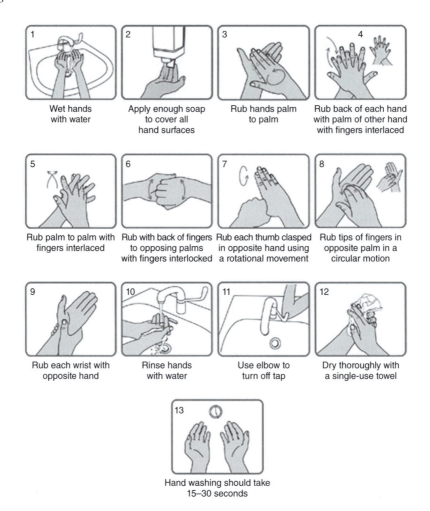

Figure 8.1: Hand washing technique with soap and water

Activity 8.3   *Reflection*

Go to one of the following sites and look at the pictures and video clips of this correct hand decontamination technique.

www.washyourhandsofthem.com/hand-hygiene–you/how-to-wash-your-hands.aspx

www.who.int/gpsc/5may/How_To_HandRub_Poster.pdf

www.powysthb.wales.nhs.uk/sitesplus/documents/1145/hand%20wash%20soap.pdf

Consider how you have decontaminated your hands and how you have seen nurses and other healthcare workers do this in your practice placements. Have you/they followed the techniques that you have seen here?

There is no answer for this activity as it involves reflecting on what you have seen and done.

You may consider that staff in practice do not always follow the detailed procedure. As a nurse in the future you will be accountable for your own practice and it is therefore important that you decontaminate your hands correctly to minimise the risk of infection and cross-infection.

Surgical hand decontamination

This is undertaken where resident flora needs to be removed from the hands. These are micro-organisms which have adapted to the acidic condition of the skin and which live in skin crevices, hair follicles and sebaceous glands. Most of these are Gram-positive bacteria. Resident flora is not easily transmitted to other people or to inanimate objects and is not removed by routine hand decontamination. However, as they do not cause infection in most situations, removing them from the skin is unnecessary. However, during more invasive procedures such as surgery there is a risk that they may enter the tissues of other people, causing infection. The aim of surgical hand decontamination is to remove/destroy transient flora and to significantly reduce resident flora on the hands. In this situation, aqueous antiseptics or surgical hand rub should be used, depending on local policy. It is currently recommended that when using an aqueous antiseptic for surgical hand decontamination, the hands should be washed for a minimum of three minutes before the first patient on the list and for two minutes between cases (Association for Perioperative Practice, 2011). Hands should be washed all the way up to the elbows. In some hospitals you may also see alcohol hand rub being used for surgical hand decontamination – this should usually be reserved for between cases in theatre as opposed to at the beginning of the list. It is recommended that when these are used they are not the general ones in use on the wards, but are those licensed specifically for surgical rubbing (Health Protection Scotland, 2015).

It has been tradition to use nail brushes to 'scrub up' in theatres (the theatre term for surgical hand decontamination), but this is no longer considered necessary. Generally nail brushes are no longer recommended in any type of hand decontamination as they become contaminated, cause abrasions on the skin and can push micro-organisms deeper into the skin and nails. If they are used in theatre they should be single use items, but there is no evidence to suggest that their use on nails decreases bacterial counts on hands (Tanner et al., 2009) (see later on Decontamination for information about single use items).

Hand decontamination agents

There are many different products available with which to perform hand hygiene including bar and liquid soap (with or without an added antiseptic), aqueous antiseptics and alcohol hand rubs.

Soap

Bar soap is not recommended for use in clinical practice. In patients' own homes when working in community settings, this may be the only soap available at the patient's hand basin. In this situation, community nurses undertake a brief risk assessment to assess whether this soap should be used or whether an alternative, such as alcohol hand rub, is appropriate. Liquid soap is what is recommended for use in most clinical areas and in most care situations when the aim is removal of transient flora. The soap does not need to contain an antiseptic agent as routine hand washing aims to remove micro-organisms from the hands rather than to kill them in-situ.

In meeting this aim there is therefore little difference in terms of liquid soaps with or without antiseptics other than possible effects on the skin.

Alcohol hand rub

As previously mentioned, these are recommended for most routine hand hygiene situation by both NICE (2012) and epic3 (Loveday et al., 2014) in both acute and primary care settings. This means that hand rubs will be used more often than liquid soap in healthcare settings. It is therefore important that staff use these correctly to ensure that they are effective in destroying transient micro-organisms (in routine hand decontamination) and resident flora (in surgical decontamination). Alcohol hand rubs have the advantage over soap in that they are quick and easy to use, can be used while walking between patients or areas so do not require nurses to stand still, require a lot less facilities, can be carried in pockets, can be used for both routine and surgical hand decontamination and are useful when facilities are lacking such as in homes. However, there can be problems in the use of hand rubs in that they are not appropriate in all situations, can sting if in contact with cuts and abrasions, can have a drying effect on skin and are flammable. One of the main considerations is incorrect use, for example, use in cases of *Clostridium difficile* when it is not effective against spores. Staff also need to wait until it has evaporated before applying gloves as this can make gloves difficult to put on and alcohol can damage the integrity of the material that gloves are made from. Because alcohol hand rubs contain emollients to minimise the drying effects, this can build up on the hands and lead to a sticky sensation. It is therefore often recommended that hands are washed every 2–3 applications of alcohol hand rub which can be problematic if moving from home to home in the community where hand washing facilities are inadequate. It is also recommended that alcohol hand rub be available at the point of care in order to improve staff compliance with hand hygiene – this was based on a Patient Safety Alert issued by the National Patient Safety Agency in 2004. Initially this was considered to be at each patient's bedside in hospital, but in some areas this led to safety concerns, particularly in paediatrics and mental health. The point of care is now therefore defined by the World Health Organization (WHO, 2009a) as the place where the patient, healthcare worker and care involving contact with the patient come together. This means that in some areas, staff keep the hand rub in small containers in their pockets so that this can be used at the point of care.

Case study

A patient was admitted to a hospital in the UK with alcohol withdrawal symptoms. He had a history of dependence on alcohol, but had not consumed any for 24 hours. During his hospital admission he was found collapsed holding a bottle of alcohol hand rub and there was another empty bottle near him. As a result of this ingestion he had to be intubated and ventilated on the intensive care unit. His blood alcohol level was found to be nine times over the legal UK driving limit, a potentially fatal level.

A Poisons Unit's database was searched and there was found to be an increase in queries from the healthcare sector about alcohol hand rubs following the NPSA recommendations. When considering whether patients intended to drink the hand rub, this was only the case in patients with alcohol dependency. Patients who ingested the hand rub unintentionally were young children, the elderly and confused patients (Archer et al., 2007).

As can be seen from this case study, access to alcohol hand rub can be dangerous for some patients and its placement in ward and care home areas therefore needs to be decided following risk assessment.

Another consequence of the widespread use and availability of alcohol hand rub was placement at hospital and ward entrances for visitors and staff to use prior to entering and leaving. In some hospitals this led to alcohol hand rub leaking onto the floor, becoming a trip hazard and the hand rub would run out at times if not replenished on a regular basis. Different healthcare organisations have dealt with this in various ways, including having drip trays under the hand rub, having replenishing schedules or even replacing hand rub at entrances with sinks and liquid soap to replace hand rub use with hand washing.

Aqueous antiseptics

These are used in surgical hand decontamination and prior to some aseptic procedures such as insertion of intravenous devices. The main antiseptics used in healthcare are triclosan, chlorhexidine gluconate and iodophors. There are differences between these chemicals in terms of their range and level of activity and their effects on the skin. Iodophors have a wider range of microbial activity than triclosan or chlorhexidine gluconate and all three have persistent chemical activity after use. Iodophors are also less affected in their activity by any organic matter on the hands. However, these can also cause more skin irritation. Triclosan causes the least skin irritation and as a consequence has been used in general hygiene products that can be bought by the general public such as soaps, tooth-pastes, disinfectant sprays and washing powder. Some NHS organisations have ceased the use of triclosan due to local resistance to it by micro-organisms such as MRSA. Due to possible skin irritation, it is not recommended that any of these products be used for routine hand decontamination.

Hand drying

Hand drying after washing is an important part of the hand hygiene process as it removes moisture and dead skin cells from the hands. Wet hands transfer micro-organisms more readily and damp hands may become chapped, increasing the risk of dry skin and therefore bacterial counts on hands. Hands that have been correctly washed can also be re-contaminated by drying if not undertaken correctly. There are three generally recognised methods of hand drying: electric hand driers, reusable cloth towels and disposable paper towels. The last of these is what is recommended in the healthcare setting and these are usually available at hand wash basins in hospitals, clinics and health centres. In patients' homes, nurses are sometimes offered a hand towel to use. This may still be referred to by some staff as a 'nurse's towel'. As with other hand washing related items in homes, a brief risk assessment is undertaken prior to use to consider what else it had been used for and if it has been laundered etc. When using alcohol hand rubs, hand drying is not required due to evaporation of the alcohol, another benefit to their use. In the operating theatre, hand drying after surgical hand decontamination is undertaken with a sterile towel to maintain asepsis (see Chapter 9).

Care of the hands

As a nurse, you decontaminate your hands multiple times each day which can have adverse effects on your skin. It is therefore important that you protect and care for your hands – after all, they are used outside of work as well as when you are in practice! Contact dermatitis is quite prevalent in healthcare workers, including nurses. It is also possible that the washing of damaged skin can lead to the shedding of increased numbers of micro-organisms which washing may then be less effective at removing. To minimise skin drying and irritation, it is important that you follow the steps as identified above, ensuring that hands are wet prior to soap application, then are rinsed and dried thoroughly when washing using soap. Hand creams should also be used frequently to protect the skin from the drying effects of soap and hand rub, though communal jars and pots of cream should be avoided. In some of your practice placements you might find wall mounted hand cream containers for use near the liquid soap and hand rub which is appropriate for use. Gloves, which are discussed later, can also have negative skin effects, so it is important to inspect skin regularly for any signs of sensitivity to glove material. Outside of the work setting, wearing gloves for activities such as washing up and gardening will help to protect the skin.

Patient hand hygiene

Patients have been implicated in outbreaks of infection and it has been identified that if both staff and patient hands are swabbed in hospitals, similar micro-organisms are identified (Landers et al., 2012). It is therefore important that the hand hygiene of patients and visitors is considered and promoted in healthcare settings, both in the hospital and primary care settings. Information and education needs to be provided to patients and carers about the importance of hand hygiene and when and how it should be performed to minimise the risk of infection and cross-infection. In the hospital setting they also need to be provided with assistance in using the available facilities, particularly if they are bed-bound and unable to reach the hand wash basin, are small children or have mental health problems which inhibit their ability to take care of their own hygiene needs. This may mean providing alternatives to soap and water such as hand wipes or hand rubs. It is particularly important to promote good hand hygiene after going to the toilet or using a commode or bedpan and before eating meals. There has been a lot of media emphasis on healthcare workers washing their hands in the NHS, but we need to ensure that patients and carers are aware that they have an important role to play, too.

The use of personal protective equipment (PPE)

PPE is worn whenever there is a risk of contact or contamination with blood, other body fluids or chemicals or potential contact with mucous membranes or breaks in the skin and includes gloves, aprons, face and eye protection, masks and gowns.

epic3 (Loveday et al., 2014) stipulates the order of removal of PPE. The guidelines state that PPE should be removed in the following order to minimise the risk of cross/self-contamination: gloves, apron, eye protection then mask. Often only gloves and an apron will be worn and in that case, the gloves should be removed followed by the apron. Prior to and following the removal of any type of PPE, hands should be decontaminated.

Gloves

These should be worn for any activity with a risk of exposure to blood or other body fluids, mucous membranes, breaks in the skin, sterile body sites, for invasive procedures and when handling sharps. The WHO (2009b) identifies when gloves should be worn and when they are not indicated (see Table 8.1). Gloves can be sterile or non-sterile and may be made from a variety of materials – which type is chosen is dependent on the activity being undertaken. Gloves are single use items, should be changed between patients and changed between different activities on the same patient to avoid moving flora from one body site to another.

Non-sterile gloves are worn to protect the staff member only – these are commonly used by nurses for a variety of activities such as obtaining blood samples, emptying urinary catheter bags and undertaking specimen collection.

Sterile gloves	Non-sterile gloves	Gloves not needed
Surgical procedures	Contact with blood, mucous	Taking blood pressure, TPR
Vaginal delivery	membranes and non-intact skin	Performing IM and SC
Aseptic procedures such as	Potential presence of highly	injections
urinary catheterisation	dangerous and infectious micro-	Transporting patients
Invasive procedures	organism	Dressing patients
Preparing TPN	Epidemic situations	Caring for eyes and ears
Preparing chemotherapy	IV insertion and removal	without secretions
agents	Obtaining a blood sample	Giving oral medications
Vascular access and	Pelvic and vaginal examinations	Placing oxygen on patient
procedures (central lines)	Suctioning non-closed circuit	
	systems	

Table 8.1: When gloves should be used – WHO recommendations (2009b)

Sterile gloves are worn for both patient and staff protection and are therefore worn for surgical procedures, for contact with sterile sites or broken skin/mucous membranes and for any aseptic procedure (see Chapter 9).

Gloves are made from material such as polythene, vinyl, natural rubber latex (NRL), neoprene and nitrile. Polythene gloves are not recommended for use in clinical practice at all and should therefore not be worn by nurses for clinical procedures. Where sterile gloves are used, it is usual for these not to be vinyl in most healthcare organisations as other materials are seen to provide better protection against blood-borne viruses than vinyl gloves, fit better and are more appropriate when a greater level of manual dexterity is needed. If the gloves required can be non-sterile, vinyl gloves can be used where there is no risk of contamination with blood. In some hospitals, vinyl gloves are only used for cleaning and not for any clinical procedures at all. This is something that you need to check with your clinical placements each time you begin in terms of the glove types available and what they recommend for use in their area for different activities.

Latex, nitrile and neoprene gloves are used in both sterile and non-sterile forms for a variety of procedures. The difference between them is in their cost and how strong they are, with latex being the cheapest of the three. In recent years there have been increasing problems in the health sector due to latex sensitivity. While latex is contained in items other than gloves, most latex exposure for nurses is related to glove use. As a consequence of this, healthcare organisations have had to undertake risk assessments related to the use of latex gloves. Some organisations have responded to this by completely removing latex gloves from their sites and replacing them with another material, such as nitrile. However, this is not the case in all settings and it remains the case that latex gloves are still the most common of the glove types due to their clinical and cost-effectiveness. It is therefore important that if you have a known latex allergy you ensure that you let your clinical placement know so that they can provide you with alternatives. It is also possible to develop a latex allergy after long-term usage – it is therefore important to look out for signs of skin irritation, breathing problems and swelling related to latex glove use.

You may have heard of nurses wearing two pairs of gloves. This is referred to as 'double gloving' and is recommended during some exposure prone procedures (EPP – see later in this chapter).

Donning and removal of gloves – The World Health Organization (WHO, 2009b) provides guidance on the donning and removal of non-sterile gloves. In the donning of gloves, the aim is to put on the glove while primarily only touching the top edge of the glove cuff near the wrist in order to minimise the risk of contaminating them and in the removal we aim not to contaminate the hands with anything on the outside of the glove. You do this in the following way.

Donning

- Take the glove from the box and put on the first glove touching only the top edge (cuff end) of the glove.
- Take the second glove from the box using your bare hand touching only the wrist end
- Put on the second glove with the gloved hand touching only the outer top edge of the second glove.

Removal

- Pinch one glove on the outer wrist edge with the other gloved hand and peel the glove off until it is inside out, without touching the bare hand or arm.
- Place the removed glove in the other gloved hand and remove the second glove by inserting the fingers of the un-gloved hand underneath the remaining glove so that the bare fingers do not touch the outside of the glove.
- The second glove should fold over the first glove and these can now be disposed of.

Where sterile gloves are concerned, removal is the same as above, but donning can seem much more complicated as the aim is to ensure that the outside of both gloves remains sterile.

Activity 8.4   *Evidence-based practice and research*

Look at one or both of the following clips. These both demonstrate the donning of sterile gloves.

www.youtube.com/watch?v=NNORa08HRjU

www.youtube.com/watch?v=UYEKrlTMnAQ

There is no answer for this activity as it involves you watching and learning from video clips.

You may consider that this looks complicated but, as with most things, it becomes easier with practice. In the theatre environment, you may see such a procedure being undertaken with the sleeves of a surgical gown pulled over the hands so that no part of the hand touches any part of the glove. It is worth your observing the donning of sterile gloves in different settings and practising until you become familiar with the correct procedures.

The wearing of gloves does not negate the need for appropriate hand hygiene. Gloves are not a complete barrier to micro-organisms; they simply minimise the contamination of the hands, and therefore hands should always be decontaminated following glove removal to ensure that micro-organisms on the hands due to small defects in the gloves or contamination during glove removal are dealt with.

Aprons

Case study

There was an outbreak of MRSA on the intensive care unit which staff were unable to explain or understand, given that the practice was one-to-one nursing so the risk of cross-infection from one patient to another within the unit was very low. On testing, the strain of MRSA was found to be the same for each of the four infected patients. One of the patients was initially known to have MRSA and had been cared for in the side room of the unit. How the MRSA had spread from this patient to three others was therefore confusing to the staff. The IPCP and consultant microbiologist came to the unit to speak to the staff in order to try to discover how cross-infection had occurred. During this visit, a physiotherapist was seen going from one patient to the next wearing the same apron. The physiotherapist was removing the gloves and decontaminating hands between patients, but not changing the apron. This was then identified as the most likely source of the cross-infection.

As can be seen from this case study, aprons can be a source of infection and cross-infection so while they may not always be seen as 'risky' when compared with gloves, for example, they can lead to serious infection if not changed between patients. Therefore, aprons should be considered single use items, be changed between different patients and between different episodes of care on the same patient, be disposed of correctly after removal (see Chapter 9) and hands should be decontaminated after each episode following removal.

As with gloves, there is a procedure for correct apron removal to avoid contaminating hands and clothing.

- Near the top of the apron with each hand at the neck, pull the apron to break the neck.
- Roll the top of the apron down over the bottom section.
- Grab the sides of the apron with each hand and pull, breaking the tie at the waist.
- Roll the apron inwards so that the outer contaminated section is on the inside.
- Dispose of appropriately.
- Decontaminate your hands.

Full body, fluid-repellent gowns

Disposable plastic aprons are the items of PPE that you will use in most nursing care situations. However, there are some circumstances where this does not provide adequate protection. When there is a risk of extensive splashing of blood or other body fluids onto your skin or clothing, you should wear a full fluid-repellent gown. This might include procedures in the operating theatre or delivery suite, or in situations where patients are spreading body fluids around the room due to, for example, mental health problems. These gowns can be disposable, so that on removal they are disposed of as waste, or non-disposable when they are disposed of in the laundry stream. The latter is often the case in the operating theatre. Whichever type they are, they should be worn as single use items.

Eye/face protection

This should be worn whenever there is a risk of splashing or contamination of the eyes or mouth. It can be considered that if there is a risk of splashing into the eyes there is also the associated risk of splashing into the mouth so full face protection, such as a face visor, might be more appropriate in most situations than eye protection only in the form of goggles. These items are often reusable so need to be decontaminated between uses. Situations when these might be used include during delivery of a baby, during some procedures in the operating theatre and during some other invasive procedures. They should also be used if masks/respiratory protection is required – see next subsection.

Masks/respiratory protection

epic3 (Loveday et al., 2014) states that appropriate respiratory protective equipment should be 'selected according to a risk assessment that takes account of the infective micro-organism, the anticipated activity and the duration of exposure'. Different types of masks are worn in the healthcare setting, dependent on whether they are used as a barrier to splashes of body fluid (when a surgical face mask is worn) or in order to protect the respiratory tract (where filtering face piece FFP respirators might be worn).

Surgical masks are single use items and are not meant to be worn for a long time. They should be changed when wet or damaged (HPA, 2012b). This type of mask does not fit tightly or mould to the face, but instead is secured behind the head by strips. There is no evidence that wearing surgical masks in the operating theatre prevents surgical site infection and you may therefore see some surgeons operating without a mask. However, these staff may then be at risk of splashing into the mouth so may need to wear a full face visor instead.

Equipment for respiratory protection needs to be able to filter out micro-organisms such as bacteria and viruses. The best level of protection is provided by an FFP3 mask and these masks need to be 'fit tested' to ensure that they correctly fit each healthcare worker and that there are no gaps around the mask. It is therefore important that, if in clinical placement you are required to wear this type of mask, you have been properly fit tested first. The masks are recommended for use in the following circumstances:

- When undertaking aerosol-producing procedures such as chest physiotherapy and bronchoscopy.

- When caring for patients with MDR-TB (multi-drug resistant tuberculosis).

- When caring for patients with pandemic influenza.

- When caring for patients with SARS (severe acute respiratory syndrome) or other acute respiratory syndromes caused by other viruses such as MERS.

- In any other situation when advised by the infection prevention and control team to do so.

Theatre head gear

There are controversies around the use of head gear in theatre and whether it contributes to reducing the risk of surgical site infection. There is no indication for wearing caps in settings outside of the operating theatre, but it is considered that, where scrubbed staff are concerned, caps reduce the dispersal of skin scales and hair into the air in the theatre and that they protect the wearer from splashes of body fluids. It is often the case, therefore, that scrubbed staff wear caps but non-scrubbed staff may not. There is also no need for theatre recovery staff to wear caps. Policies differ between organisations so if you are ever on placement in a theatre setting it is worth checking their local procedures regarding cap use and their rationale for their procedure. It is generally local policy not to wear theatre clothing outside of the theatre department.

Sharps management

In 2010 European employment ministers agreed a directive aimed at preventing sharps injuries in healthcare settings. This became UK law in May 2013 in the form of The Health and Safety (Sharps Instruments in Health Care) Regulations 2013. While these regulations place responsibilities on employers, those practising using sharps such as nurses need to control risks by practising safely, including the following:

- Not resheathing or recapping needles.

- Not bending or breaking needles.

- Disposing of sharps immediately after use.

- Wearing gloves when using sharps (while these cannot prevent injury, there is evidence that the glove can remove a significant proportion of blood from a needle prior to it entering the skin during an injury).

- Disposing of needles/sharps and syringes/holders as one unit rather than disassembling after use and prior to disposal.

- Not passing sharps directly from hand to hand.

- Keeping sharps handling to a minimum.

- Using safer sharps devices where these are available and provided (RCN, 2013a).

Surgical blade/scalpel use

You might consider that outside of theatre, blades will not be used, but this is not the case. In clinical practice, blades are used for various procedures including in some aspects of wound management and suture removal (where a specific type of blade is used). It is therefore important that you familiarise yourself with these items as they may appear different in various organisations. For example, the scalpel and holder may be one unit which is disposed of after use, or it may be a safety scalpel where the blade is retracted back into the holder then disposed of as one unit after use. In other areas, the blade may need to be attached to and removed from a reusable holder. Great care should be taken with these items and you should ensure that you are fully competent in their use before dealing with them. Some areas may use a blade remover in these cases whereas others may use forceps. The best option in terms of safety is either a safety scalpel or a scalpel and holder which are built as one unit. The Association for Perioperative Practitioners provides advice on safe handling for different types of blade/scalpel.

Sharps disposal and sharps bins

It is essential that sharps including items such as needles, blades and suture cutters are disposed of safely in the appropriate containers which have been correctly assembled to prevent injuries to staff and others. All sharps should be disposed of immediately after use and at the point of use which essentially means that wherever a sharp is being used, a sharps bin should be available. So, for example, if in a patient's house giving an injection or obtaining a blood sample, a sharps bin should be taken into the house. In hospitals it is now common to have procedure trays with bins attached so that all the items required for the procedure, including the sharps bin, can be taken to the bedside. These trays facilitate safe disposal and good practice.

You may find in some areas of practice that sharps bins are delivered ready assembled. However, in other areas they will need to be assembled, that is, the lid will need to be securely fastened to the container. It is therefore important that you are aware of how to do this for each type of container, as different manufacturers produce different bins and lids. For example, some require each corner of the lid to click into place whereas others have a round lid which needs to be secured all the way around. Sharps bins also have labels which need to be completed by the staff assembling them and the staff seal them once the contents have reached the fill-line. These need to be completed to provide an audit trail. When in use, sharps bins should be kept out of reach of vulnerable people, such as children, and the temporary seal on the lid should be utilised to avoid access to the sharps in the bin.

> ### Case study
>
> *In a GP surgery a GP was undertaking a clinic where they were seeing babies and administering injections. A mother had brought her baby to the clinic, along with her three-year-old daughter. During the consultation with the GP, the three-year-old was attracted to a yellow bin which was on the floor. The temporary seal was not in use and the child put her hand into the bin, sustaining a needlestick injury. This incident was investigated by the Health and Safety Executive and the GP was prosecuted for unsafe practice. In this situation, not only was the bin on the floor and therefore accessible to vulnerable children, but the temporary seal was also not in use. The child had to undertake blood tests for several months afterwards to ensure that she had not been infected with a blood-borne virus.*

As can be seen from the above scenario, position and use of sharps bins can be a safety issue and as nurses we need to ensure that we follow the correct procedures.

Management of a sharps/needlestick injury

Unfortunately, injuries do occur, whether from poor practice, incorrect disposal or through no fault of the healthcare worker, such as the patient moving or behaving in an unexpected way during use of the sharp. It is therefore important that nurses are aware of the correct procedure following such events, in order to protect themselves from infection. A survey undertaken by the Royal College of Nursing in 2008 (RCN, 2009) found that around half of nurses had received a needlestick injury from a needle that had been used on a patient so this is clearly an important area of practice.

Sharps injuries from items contaminated with blood or other body fluids are referred to as 'percutaneous exposure' as the healthcare worker's skin is cut or penetrated by the sharp. This is different to 'mucocutaneous exposure' which occurs when areas such as the eyes, mouth or inside of the nose or an open wound are contaminated by blood or another body fluid. Transmissions of blood-borne viruses to healthcare workers, including hepatitis B and C and HIV, have all been as a result of percutaneous exposure (HPA, 2012). While prevention of injuries and exposure through best practice is the best approach, the correct management of injuries also helps to minimise infection risk. When considering the main blood-borne viruses, the HPA (2012) identifies the risk of infection from a contaminated needle to be one in three for hepatitis B, one in 30 for hepatitis C and one in 300 for HIV.

> ### Case study
>
> *Susan is a 48-year-old nurse who works in a community mental health setting. She is referred to the IPC practitioner and occupational health department as she has been newly diagnosed with hepatitis B and needs advice about living with the virus and how this may impact on her nursing role. During discussions with the IPC nurse, Susan admits that she was offered immunisation against hepatitis B by the*
>
> *(Continued)*

continued . . .

non-NHS organisation that she works for, but declined the offer as she felt she was not at risk. She considered her role as a mental health nurse to be a mainly non-patient-contact role. However, she also admitted that over the previous year she had sustained three sharps injuries from needles used to administer depot injections to her patient group. Following these incidents she had not followed first aid procedures, had not completed any accident or incident forms, had not informed her manager and had not contacted occupational health for any follow-up. Again, she considered that the injuries were low risk and had the view that 'it wouldn't happen to her'. Although it could not be confirmed that any of these injuries was responsible for her hepatitis B infection, it is possible that one of these injuries, the fact that she did not act or report on them, and her decision not to be immunised resulted in the infection.

As can be seen from the case study above, the proper management of sharps injuries is important for healthcare workers to reduce their risk of being infected with blood-borne viruses. One of the documented reasons for poor compliance with sharps management procedures is that staff do not see the risks associated with poor practice and consider that it 'won't happen' to them. This is not the case and staff have been infected with blood-borne viruses. The correct procedure to follow is found in policies and procedures and on posters on walls in healthcare settings. The main points are:

- Encourage the area to bleed.
- Wash the area.
- Cover with a waterproof dressing.
- Complete an incident/accident form.
- Contact occupational health or A&E outside of normal working hours.
- Inform the university.

It is important that you follow these steps to minimise the risks to yourself, to prevent future injuries and to ensure that you receive any follow-up care required, such as hepatitis B booster injections, even if you are a non-responder to the initial course of vaccine.

Exposure prone procedures (EPP) and blood-borne virus (BBV) in infected healthcare workers

EPPs are those invasive procedures where there is a risk that injury to the worker may result in exposure of the patient's open tissues to the blood of the worker. These include procedures where the worker's gloved hands may be in contact with sharp instruments, needle tips or sharp tissues (e.g. spicules of bone or teeth) inside a patient's open body cavity, wound or confined anatomical space where the hands or fingertips may not be completely visible at all times. Such procedures occur mainly in surgery, obstetrics and gynaecology, dentistry and some aspects of midwifery. Most clinical duties do not involve EPPs; exceptions include accident and emergency and theatre nursing.
(Public Health England, 2014)

There is guidance available from Public Health England (2014) for the NHS in managing health-care workers infected with a BBV, including HIV, who perform EPPs. Any healthcare workers with a BBV, whether they undertake EPPs or not, should be managed via occupational health to ensure that any risks to both them and others are minimised.

Decontamination

As a word, decontamination could mean one of three different processes – namely cleaning, disinfection or sterilisation. Therefore when asked to decontaminate something as a nurse, you need to know specifically which process is required. According to the Health and Safety Executive, 'decontamination is a combination of processes that removes or destroys contamination so that infectious agents or other contaminants cannot reach a susceptible site in sufficient quantities to initiate infection, or other harmful response.' We therefore decontaminate items to reduce cross-infection from medical equipment or the environment to people, such as staff, patients and visitors.

The choice of process should be based on a risk assessment of what the piece of equipment or device is used for.

Cleaning

Cleaning physically removes contamination, including some micro-organisms and, if soiling is present, it is an essential step before effective disinfection or sterilisation can be performed. Cleaning does not necessarily destroy all micro-organisms. It is generally undertaken using detergent and warm water, but detergent-based wipes can be used on items which cannot be exposed to water. Cleaning is generally undertaken on low-risk items such as those that are not in contact with the patient or items in contact with healthy intact skin which are not contaminated with any blood or other body fluids. Low-risk items might include drip stands, floors, examination couches, bed mattresses, hoists and blood pressure cuffs, as long as they are not contaminated with body fluids.

Wherever practical, automated processes for cleaning are preferable to manual processes and this type of cleaning is carried out in some departments by washer-disinfectors. However, for general ward cleaning this is not practical. Wherever possible, cleaning of equipment should be carried out in a designated 'dirty' area. In some hospitals, large items such as beds are sent to specific departments for cleaning by automated processes. When cleaning equipment you should wear the appropriate PPE and follow manufacturer's instructions for the detergent or wipe being used.

Cleanliness of both equipment and the environment is a part of the Health and Social Care Act Code of Practice (DH, 2015). There are national specifications for cleanliness in the NHS which provides 49 element standards for both cleaning and cleaning surfaces within the NHS. The standards relate to visible cleanliness so that all parts of a particular item are free from dust, dirt, blood etc. There is also a national colour coding scheme for equipment used for cleaning (NPSA, 2007) which identifies the colours of aprons, cloths, buckets and mop handles to be used in different areas. You need to ensure that the colour coding system within your placement area is adhered to as while this was recommended, not all areas have adapted this particular system. The NPSA (2007) recommendations were as follows:

- Red for bathrooms, showers, sinks, toilets and floors.
- Blue for general areas such as offices.
- Green for catering areas including ward kitchens.
- Yellow for isolation areas.

In some circumstances, a procedure known as a 'deep clean' is undertaken. This might be of an isolation room following the discharge of a patient with *Clostridium difficile*, for example. This might involve more advanced systems such as steam cleaning, light sources such as UV light or the use of hydrogen peroxide vapour (HPV). A deep clean involves removing curtains and cleaning walls and air vents in addition to the usual patient equipment and floors.

In addition to the cleaning of equipment and medical devices, as nurses we have to consider the provision of a safe environment for our patients which means ensuring that it is clean. epic3 (Loveday et al., 2014) highlights the need for the hospital environment to be visibly clean, free from dust and dirt and acceptable to staff, patients and visitors. It also provides recommendations related to the cleaning of equipment for shared patient use between uses and increasing cleaning levels in the case of some infections.

Disinfection

The aim of disinfection is to reduce the number of micro-organisms present to a level that is unlikely to cause infection. Disinfection may destroy or inactivate many or all pathogenic micro-organisms, but not spores and not some viruses. The efficacy of disinfection is dependent on the number of micro-organisms initially present which is why cleaning is an essential prerequisite to effective disinfection, as previously mentioned. Disinfection should be carried out on medium/moderate-risk items, though some items which would appear to be medium risk are not appropriate for disinfection, such as vaginal speculae, as disinfection does not destroy all of the viruses which may be present in the vagina of some women. Medium-risk items are generally items in contact with mucous membranes or low-risk items contaminated with body fluids. Such items might include reusable bed pans, oral thermometers, **auriscope** ear pieces and so on. Disinfection can be undertaken using chemical disinfectants or by the use of heat. Chemical disinfectants used on tissue, such as the skin, are known as antiseptics. Whenever using disinfectants, you should consider the following points:

- Follow the manufacturer's instructions for both the disinfectant and the items being disinfected to ensure that they are compatible with each other and that any special precautions required are taken.
- If making up a disinfectant by adding water (such as to tablets), the made-up solution should usually be discarded after 24 hours as some disinfectants can become unstable after this time and/or lose their level of activity.
- Follow any special instructions such as wearing PPE, opening windows etc. according to manufacturer's instructions.
- Take care when using disinfectant sprays as there is a risk of inhaling the disinfectant and you may not cover the whole area to be disinfected with the spray.

There are many disinfectants available, both in healthcare and in domestic situations. Some of the commonly used chemicals in healthcare include sodium hypochlorite (chlorine-releasing agents), alcohol (as wipes or liquid) and ammonium compounds. These have varying levels of efficacy against different micro-organisms and both appropriate and inappropriate uses. There has also been recent debate about chlorine and chlorine dioxide-based cleaning which may mean that some organisations are now limiting use or not using these at all.

- *Chlorine-releasing agents* – these are often used where there is blood contamination as it has good activity against BBVs. However, it should not be used to soak metal items as it corrodes metal and it should be used in well ventilated areas.

- *Alcohol* – this can be used on metal items, but it not recommended for use on thin rubber or plastic as it damages their integrity. Problems have been caused in the past by indiscriminate use of alcohol-based wipes on items such as bed mattresses and baby changing mattresses where they have damaged the covering and allowed body fluids to contaminate the foam underneath.

- *Ammonium compounds* – these are not widely used by nurses in the healthcare setting as they have a limited use against infections in healthcare. They are most often used in the home setting.

In addition to these, high level disinfectants are used on some equipment such as **endoscopes**.

Sterilisation

Sterilisation destroys all micro-organisms, including spores, but is not effective against prions. Sterilisation is undertaken using heat in an autoclave – this may be on-site, such as the use of a bench-top steriliser in a dental or GP practice, or off-site, such as in a central sterile services department within a hospital. This process is carried out on high-risk items such as surgical instruments and other items inserted into sterile body cavities or in contact with broken skin or broken mucous membranes. Some items which require sterilisation are destroyed by heat, such as flexible endoscopes, so these are decontaminated using a high level disinfectant.

Single use

Items designated as single use by a manufacturer should be used once and then be disposed of. The re-use of items designated as single use has implications not just in relation to IPC, but also related to safety and effectiveness and also has legal implications. Items designated single use by the manufacturer have the symbol shown in Figure 8.2 on their packaging.

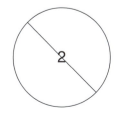

Figure 8.2: Symbol on the packaging of items designated for single use

Single use items include things such as gloves and aprons, needles, syringes, thermometer ear pieces and so on and should not be confused with single patient use items referred to later.

Activity 8.5   *Evidence-based practice and research*

The next time you are in placement, have a look at some of the items in the treatment room and the store cupboard and identify the items which have the single use symbol on them. Did you know that all of these items should only be used once? Have you seen any of these items being used more than once?

There is no answer for this activity as it involves you observing in practice.

Single patient use

These items can be reused on the same patient multiple times, but not be used on anyone else. Once they are not being used by the patient, such as following discharge from hospital or after death, the items should be disposed of as waste. Such items need to be decontaminated according to manufacturer instructions and may include things such as nebuliser masks and oxygen tubing.

Laundry management

In hospitals in particular, there are systems in place for laundry/linen processing such as sheets and pillow cases, towels, blankets and curtains. Clean linen is usually stored in designated areas which are for clean linen only. This area should not be used for the storage of used or soiled linen or other items.

When you are likely to need to place used linen into a bag or suitable container for reprocessing within the hospital setting, you should ensure that such a container is available as close as possible to the point of use so that the linen is not placed onto the floor or other surface such as a bedside table, or that it is not carried in the hands of staff to another location for disposal. When removing items such as sheets from beds for washing, you should not shake these prior to placing into the linen receptacle as this may promote the spread of dust, skin scales and bacterial spores throughout the environment. Laundry bags should not be overfilled and should not be used for the disposal of other items. These bags go to the laundry department or to an off-site laundry for processing and injuries can be caused to laundry staff by items incorrectly disposed of such as instruments and sharps. Once used linen has been disposed of into the appropriate linen bag it should not then be removed. You will find that in many hospitals linen bags are generally white but this may differ between organisations. The most up-to-date guidance on linen categories is as follows (DH, 2013):

- *Used (soiled and fouled) linen* – This definition applies to all used linen, irrespective of state, but on occasions contaminated by body fluids or blood. It does not apply to linen from infectious patients; those suspected of being infectious; and other linen covered by the following paragraph 'infectious linen'.

- *Infectious linen* – This definition applies to linen from patients with diarrhoea; linen contaminated with blood or body fluids from patients with blood-borne viruses; other conditions as specified by local policy. Linen from patients infected with, or at high risk of having, hazard group 4 organisms (haemorraghic fever viruses such as Lassa fever) should not be returned to a laundry.

- *Heat labile items* – This category includes fabrics damaged by the normal heat disinfection process and those likely to be damaged at thermal disinfection temperatures. These fabrics should be washed at the highest temperature possible for the item; disinfection may be achieved by chemical disinfection, if required.

You will find that red water soluble bags are used in most healthcare organisations for infectious linen which is then placed inside a white laundry bag.

Management of blood and body fluid spillages

There is the potential for blood and body fluid spillages to transmit blood-borne viruses such as hepatitis B. Where such a spillage occurs, it is important that they are dealt with immediately to reduce risks to staff, patients and visitors. Different healthcare organisations have different policies and procedures for this issue so it is worth checking with your practice placements what to do in case of a spillage.

If there is a blood or spillage of other body fluids, PPE should be worn to deal with it. If the spillage is on a soft furnishing such as an upholstered chair or carpet, you may need to discuss this with the IPCP so that he/she can advise you on what to do next. In cases of severe contamination, upholstered items may need to be destroyed.

If the spill is on a surface such as a vinyl floor, the next action is dependent on the body fluid. Spillages which only contain urine, faeces or vomit should be soaked up using disposable paper towels. In some areas, gelling agents are used for urine spillages. Following removal of the spillage, the area should be decontaminated with a chlorine-releasing agent such as sodium hypochlorite containing 1000 parts per million (PPM) of available chlorine. In some areas, this second step is not undertaken and the area is just cleaned with detergent. If the body fluid spilled is blood, breast milk, cerebrospinal fluid, peritoneal, pleural, synovial or amniotic fluid, semen or a vaginal secretion, a chlorine-releasing agent should be used. In some areas, such as operating theatres, chlorine-releasing granules are used to cover the spill for three minutes and then the waste is disposed of. If granules are not in use in that particular area, disposable paper towels should be placed over the spill and a chlorine-releasing solution with 10,000 ppm of available chlorine should be poured onto it, left for three minutes and then waste be discarded including PPE.

Compliance with IPC precautions and barriers to good practice

Despite the knowledge that we have about infection and the precautions we can implement to reduce the risk of infection and cross-infection, healthcare staff do not always do what they should. By this, we mean that staff do not comply 100% of the time with standard precautions. For example, they do not always wash their hands when they should or change their gloves when they should. This has been investigated in many areas of practice across the world and the general finding is that compliance can be low in all professions. There may be many reasons for this and factors that stop people complying (Darawad and Al-Hussami, 2013; Tada et al., 2015), including a lack of time, lack of knowledge, attitudes, lack of facilities, poor habits and so on. Compliance can be poor with both standard and transmission based precautions, even in areas such as A&E and the operating theatre (Chan, 2010; Russell et al., 2014) which are often seen as higher risk areas for patients in terms of infection.

Activity 8.6 — Reflection

Think about your previous practice placements. When staff have not complied with IPC precautions 100% of the time, what do you think has been the reason for this? What has stopped them complying? If you have not yet had a clinical placement, what reasons do you think staff might give for not complying? You may find the answer to this question by undertaking a quick literature search and identifying journal articles based on research about compliance in IPC.

Suggested reasons can be found at the end of this chapter.

You may have identified several reasons, but you need to consider whether these are real barriers to good practice. Part of the nursing role is in the identification of barriers and working to overcome these. Considering why people do not decontaminate their hands, for example, and considering what we can do to address this improves standards of care and, in turn, patient outcomes in relation to infection. Rather than accepting barriers to good practice and continuing to say 'we cannot do this because . . .' we need to work to address barriers and improve practice. Bad practice is not acceptable practice and should never be considered normal in practice placements because of perceived barriers. Part of the NMC Code (2015) and the NMC Essential Skills Clusters (2010) highlight that nurses need to identify and challenge poor practice in others – this is particularly relevant in IPC where patients' lives may be at risk if we do not do what we can to prevent infection. There is now increasing focus on what are termed 'human factors' which need to be addressed to improve compliance and patient safety, with the definition from the International Ergonomics Association Council being 'Ergonomics (or human factors) is the scientific discipline concerned with understanding of interactions among humans and other elements of a system and the profession that applies theory, principles, data and methods to design in order to optimise human well-being and overall system performance' (Storr et al., 2013). This highlights the complexities inherent in improving compliance and overcoming barriers to good practice plus mitigating for human error.

Activity 8.7 — Multiple choice questions

1. What is the most appropriate method to decontaminate physically soiled hands?

   a) Use an alcohol hand gel
   b) Wash hands with soap and water
   c) Wash hands with a disinfectant soap

    d)   Wash hands with soap and water and then use an alcohol hand gel

    e)   Use an alcohol hand gel and then wash hands with a disinfectant

2. What is the most appropriate method to decontaminate hands when caring for patients suffering *Clostridium difficile* infection?

    a)   Use an alcohol hand gel following patient contact

    b)   Wash hands with soap and water following patient contact

    c)   Wash hands with a disinfectant following patient contact

    d)   Wash hands with soap and water and then use an alcohol hand gel following patient contact

    e)   Use an alcohol hand gel and then wash hands with a disinfectant following patient contact

3. What method of decontamination is used for low-risk items?

    a)   Disinfection

    b)   Single use

    c)   Single patient use

    d)   Cleaning

    e)   Sterilisation

4. When making up disinfectants by adding water, after how long should the solution made be thrown away?

    a)   2 days

    b)   1 week

    c)   12 hours

    d)   24 hours

    e)   1 month

5. What type of organism does sterilisation not destroy?

    a)   Bacteria

    b)   Viruses

    c)   Fungi

    d)   Prions

    e)   Parasites

6. What hand decontamination agent should be used for removing transient flora?

    a)   An aqueous antiseptic

    b)   Soap and water

    c)   Soap and water followed by alcohol hand rub

    d)   Soap and water followed by aqueous antiseptic

    e)   Aqueous antiseptic followed by alcohol hand rub

(Continued)

continued . . .

7. In which of the following situations can alcohol hand rub be used?

   a) When patients have *Clostridium difficile*
   b) When hands are visibly soiled with blood
   c) Before aseptic procedures when hands are visibly clean
   d) When hands are visibly soiled with urine
   e) For a surgical scrub on the first case in theatre

8. In which situation is the removal of resident flora important?

   a) Before undertaking catheter care
   b) Before undertaking surgical procedures
   c) After any patient care activity
   d) After removing an intravenous device
   e) Before obtaining a routine blood sample

9. Items in contact with intact mucous membranes are considered, in terms of decontamination risks, to be:

   a) Low-risk
   b) Medium-risk
   c) High-risk
   d) Very high-risk
   e) No risk at all

10. What is the immediate management of a sharps injury?

   a) Wash with antiseptic and cover
   b) Cover it and report it
   c) Wash it, cover it, report it
   d) Encourage bleeding, cover it, report it
   e) Encourage bleeding, wash it, cover it, report it

Chapter summary

In this chapter we have looked at standard infection prevention and control precautions which are used in healthcare settings to prevent infection and cross-infection. You should now have more knowledge and understanding of these precautions and how they apply to your clinical practice as a nurse. In the next chapter we will take this further by focusing on additional IPC related precautions, including those which are transmission based.

Activities: Brief outline answers

Activity 8.1: Evidence-based practice and research (page 121)

The WHO five moments for hand hygiene:

1. Before touching a patient
2. Before clean/aseptic procedures
3. After body fluid exposure risk
4. After touching a patient
5. After touching a patient's surroundings

Activity 8.6: Reflection (page 142)

Reasons for non-compliance with IPC precautions might have included the following, but this is not an exhaustive list:

- Cost
- Lack of knowledge/education/policies
- Workload
- Time
- Lack of leadership/management support/role models
- Lack of appropriate facilities/poor access to facilities
- Skin reactions
- Risk perception
- Lack of motivation
- Staffing levels
- Too busy
- Job demands
- Poor habits
- Stress
- Conflict of interest, e.g. patient doesn't like staff wearing PPE
- Interferes with manual dexterity (gloves)
- Forgot to do it
- Poor communication

Activity 8.7: MCQs (pages 142–4)

1. What is the most appropriate method to decontaminate physically soiled hands?

   b)   Wash hands with soap and water

2. What is the most appropriate method to decontaminate hands when caring for patients suffering *Clostridium difficile* infection?

   b)   Wash hands with soap and water following patient contact

3. What method of decontamination is used for low risk items?

   d)   Cleaning

4. When making up disinfectants by adding water, after how long should the solution made be thrown away?

   d)   24 hours

5. What type of organism does sterilisation not destroy?

   d)   Prions

6. What hand decontamination agent should be used for removing transient flora?

   b)   Soap and water

7. In which of the following situations can alcohol hand rub be used?

   c)   Before aseptic procedures when hands are visibly clean

8. In which situation is the removal of resident flora important?

   b)   Before undertaking surgical procedures

9. Items in contact with intact mucous membranes are considered, in terms of decontamination risks, to be:

   b)   Medium-risk

10. What is the immediate management of a sharps injury?

    e)   Encourage bleeding, wash it, cover it, report it

Further reading

Health Protection Scotland (2015) *National Infection Prevention and Control Manual.* HPS.

This document is freely available online, even outside of Scotland, and has been produced to guide the NHS in Scotland in writing their own policies relating to IPC.

PHE (2014) *The management of HIV infected healthcare workers who perform exposure prone procedures: updated guidance, January 2014.* London: PHE.

This document contains full and detailed information about this specific group of staff.

RCN (2013) *Sharps safety. RCN guidance to support the implementation of The Health and Safety (Sharps Instruments in Healthcare Regulations) 2013.* London: RCN.

This provides more comprehensive information about how to implement the regulations in healthcare settings in the UK and might be useful for assignments related to sharps safety.

Weston, D (2013) *Fundamentals of Infection Prevention and Control: Theory and Practice.* Chichester: Wiley-Blackwell.

This book provides further information about standard IPC precautions for those students who want a more in-depth knowledge and understanding of issues such as donning and removing sterile gloves.

Useful websites

http://cks.nice.org.uk

This is the part of the NICE website which contains clinical summaries for topics in an A–Z format including different infections. This includes aspects such as BBV-infected healthcare workers.

www.documents.hps.scot.nhs.uk/hai/infection-control/ic-manual/ipcm-p-v2.4.pdf

This is a link to the HPS infection control manual which provides information on infections in Appendix 14 for which transmission based precautions should be applied in addition to standard precautions.

Chapter 9
Other infection prevention and control precautions

....

NMC Standards for Pre-registration Nursing Education

This chapter will address the following competencies:

Domain 3: Nursing practice and decision-making

Generic competencies

4.1 Adult nurses must safely use invasive and non-invasive procedures, medical devices, and current technological and pharmacological interventions, where relevant, in medical and surgical nursing practice, providing information and taking account of individual needs and preferences.

6. All nurses must practice safely by being aware of the correct use, limitations and hazards of common interventions, including nursing activities, treatments, and the use of medical devices and equipment. The nurse must be able to evaluate their use, report any concerns promptly through appropriate channels and modify care where necessary to promote safety. They must contribute to the collection of local and national data and formulation of policy on risks, hazards and adverse outcomes.

....

....

NMC Essential Skills Clusters: Infection Control

This chapter will address the following competences within this cluster:

*   Adheres to local policy and national guidelines on dress code for prevention and control of infection, including: footwear, hair, piercing and nails (Progression point 1).
*   Maintains a high standard of personal hygiene (Progression point 1).
*   Wears appropriate clothing for the care delivered in all environments (Progression point 1).
*   Demonstrates understanding of the principles of wound management, healing and asepsis. Safely performs basic wound care using clean and aseptic techniques in a variety of settings (Progression point 2).
*   Safely delivers care under supervision to people who require to be nursed in isolation or in protective isolation settings (Progression point 2).

(Continued)

....

continued . . .

- Adheres to health and safety at work legislation and infection control policies regarding the safe disposal of all waste, soiled linen, blood and other body fluids and disposing of 'sharps' including in the home setting (Progression point 2).
- Manages hazardous waste and spillages in accordance with local health and safety policies (Progression point 3).
- Applies a range of appropriate measures to prevent infection including application of safe and effective aseptic technique (Progression point 3).
- Safely performs wound care, applying non-touch or aseptic techniques in a variety of settings (Progression point 3).
- Assesses the needs of the infectious person, or people and applies appropriate isolation techniques (Progression point 3).
- Identifies suitable alternatives when isolation facilities are unavailable and principles have to be applied in unplanned circumstances (Progression point 3).
- Adheres to infection prevention and control policies and procedures at all times and ensures that colleagues work according to good practice guidelines (Progression point 3).
- Manages overall environment to minimise risk (Progression point 3).

Chapter aims

After reading this chapter, you will be able to:

- Identify the different types of isolation.
- Describe options available if single rooms are not free to use.
- Describe the precautions which should be applied to patients in isolation.
- Identify the different categories of waste and how these should be disposed of.
- Discuss the basis for uniform recommendations from the DH.
- Identify the elements of an appropriate uniform in healthcare.
- Identify the different types of asepsis.
- Identify some of the clinical skills to which principles of asepsis should be applied.

In the previous chapter we considered IPC precautions which are considered to be 'standard' in that they are applied to all patients, whether known to have an infection or not. In addition to these, there are some precautions which are not considered as standard and which might be applied in some situations with some patients but not with others. Some of these precautions will be discussed in this chapter. Firstly we will discuss isolation and how this might be applied in practice, including different types of isolation. We will then consider waste management, in particular waste segregation and colour coding requirements in healthcare settings. Uniform policies with specific reference to Department of Health recommendations will then be discussed followed by a look at the principles of asepsis and when these should be applied. Throughout the chapter are scenarios, case studies and activities to enable you to apply the knowledge gained to practice settings and to test what you have learned.

Patient isolation

Patients may be isolated in healthcare for a variety of reasons, not all related to infection. For example, to provide privacy and dignity to dying patients, to isolate noisy or disruptive patients from others and as a previous form of treatment in mental health settings (known as the 'seclusion room'). Where patients are isolated for IPC reasons, this is divided into two types of isolation: source isolation (previously referred to as barrier nursing) where patients with infections are isolated to protect others; and protective isolation (formerly known as reverse barrier nursing) where patients are isolated to protect themselves from getting infections from others. Isolation is one of the transmission based precautions referred to in the previous chapter which may be applied to some patients, in addition to standard precautions, due to transmission by the contact, droplet or airborne route.

Source isolation

This type of isolation basically isolates the source of infection, that is, the patient, in order to minimise the risk of transmission of this infection to others. This may be a confirmed infection or one which is suspected, such as in the case of diarrhoea and vomiting of an unknown cause, until this suspicion is either confirmed or refuted. There are some infections for which patients will usually be isolated regardless of the hospital where you have your placement. With other infections, there may be local variations dependent on the infection, how prevalent it is, what type of ward the patient has been admitted to and availability of isolation facilities. For example, in some areas of the country, all patients with MRSA will be isolated but in others, they will only be isolated under specific conditions, such as site of infection or admission to a high-risk area such as vascular surgery. This can be confusing for students who may have placements in a variety of different hospitals, sometimes across different towns or cities. You therefore need to familiarise yourself with isolation policies in different organisations as you start each placement.

When patients are in source isolation, the usual standard infection prevention and control precautions should be applied as discussed in the previous chapter. Transmission based precautions may also be required, such as airborne precautions and the use of masks for some patients. Adequate supplies of PPE should be provided, ideally outside the isolation room so that these can be donned prior to entering the room. Ideally isolation rooms should have their own en-suite facilities, but this is not always the case. At a minimum, however, there should be a hand basin for hand washing to be undertaken. PPE should be removed and hands decontaminated prior to leaving the room.

It may or may not have crossed your mind at this point that if a patient has an infection, in particular one which is transmitted by an airborne route, and they are placed into a single room, whenever the door to that room is opened, the air from the room will escape into the surrounding environment, such as a main ward or corridor. This means that micro-organisms could then 'escape' from the room and be a potential source of infection to others. In most cases of source isolation, this is not a serious risk, but there are some infections for which it is a risk. In these cases, patients may need to be nursed in specialist isolation room (such as a negative pressure room). These include patients with infections such as viral haemorrhagic fevers (e.g. Ebola), multi-drug resistant tuberculosis

(MDR-TB), SARS, MERS and H5N1 influenza. Most such patients will be cared for in designated infectious diseases units which can be found in some NHS Trusts within the UK.

Cohort nursing

The Health and Social Care Act Code of Practice (DH, 2015) highlights that organisations, such as hospitals, which provide in-patient care, should have the ability to provide, or secure such provision of, adequate isolation facilities. Allocation of isolation facilities should also be based on local risk assessment. It is unfortunately the case, however, that many hospitals do not have enough single rooms to meet the need at certain times, particularly when there are other reasons outside of IPC for the use of single rooms. In these cases, cohort nursing can be applied to some infections after consultation with the IPCT. This means that several patients with the same infection are nursed together in the same place, such as a six-bedded room. This can be applied to many infections such as norovirus, MRSA, *Clostridium difficile*, chicken pox and so on. However, there are some cases where cohort nursing SHOULD NOT be applied. Patients with pulmonary TB, for example, should not be nursed together due to differing antimicrobial resistance patterns. Patients with diarrhoea and vomiting of an unknown cause should not be isolated together in case the cause is more than one micro-organism, such as in the case study below.

Case study

The community infection control practitioner was called one Friday afternoon by the local hospital's consultant microbiologist to assist in an outbreak as the hospital IPCP was on leave while another was off sick. On arrival at the hospital, the IPCP found that four wards had outbreaks of diarrhoea and vomiting. Following the provision of advice about closing the wards to admissions and transfers and only discharging fit patients to their own homes, the IPCP discussed IPC measures with the nursing staff. As the IPCP was not involved in any on-call rota for IPC advice, she next reviewed the situation the following Monday. At this point a further two wards were affected and another hospital in the same town reported two wards with similar outbreaks. Later that day she received a call from a local nursing home reporting six residents with diarrhoea and vomiting. On investigation, the following was identified:

- *Despite advice to the contrary, one of the initially affected wards had discharged an affected patient to the nursing home which had led to an outbreak there.*
- *Two patients had also been transferred from the affected wards to the other hospital, had subsequently developed symptoms and then an outbreak had ensued.*
- *Patients with diarrhoea and vomiting, the cause of which was not known at that point, were all placed in bays together in order to apply cohort nursing.*

It was subsequently discovered that some of the patients had norovirus, whereas others had Clostridium difficile which meant that they should not have been in the same room.

As a result of cohorting, transferring and discharging inappropriately, a total of eight wards and a nursing home were closed.

Activity 9.1   *Reflection/evidence-based practice*

Consider the above case study. What things do you think could have been done differently to minimise the impact of the outbreak of infection? If you are currently in clinical placement, discuss this with one of the nurses and highlight how this would have been managed in the placement area, and what factors might have prevented good management.

Suggested thinking points can be found at the end of the chapter.

As can be seen from the scenario and activity, mistakes made had a significant impact on patients and the wards, but there can be difficulties in applying isolation which may have been highlighted by the activity. It is also worth noting that some areas have access to on-call IPCN/Ps but others do not.

Where CPE is concerned, if the specific organism is known, patients with the same specific organism (such as *Klebsiella*, for example) can be nursed together. However, if the only information is that four patients have CPE but you are unaware of the specific micro-organism/strain, these should not be nursed together. This is because you may have a patient with *Klebsiella*, one with *E. coli* and so on – basically not the same infection but all grouped as CPE (see Chapter 3).

Unfortunately within healthcare organisations we cannot always isolate or cohort patients as needed due to a lack of resources, in particular single rooms or small bays that may need to have empty beds to cohort a small number of patients. This means that there are occasions when patients who are infected or colonised with an organism who should be isolated may have to be nursed in a bay with patients who are not infected or colonised. In these situations, the strict application of IPC precautions is vital as is close liaison with the IPC team, nurse managers and bed managers. This can often occur with patients with MRSA colonisation. In such cases, the risks to surrounding patients need to be considered so that those with invasive devices such as urinary catheters are not in a bed next to a patient with MRSA, for example. The measures required should be based on a risk assessment which takes into account the nature and severity of the infection, the needs of the individual patient and the susceptibility of other patients in the ward, unit or department. Many healthcare organisations now have reporting systems in place related to adverse incident reporting which are used when a patient needs to be isolated but there are no facilities available to do so. In most organisations, infections transmitted by the airborne route are prioritised for single room isolation above those by the contact or faecal–oral routes.

In some areas, isolation is rarely practical as there may be no isolation rooms and it may not be appropriate to transfer the patient to another ward or department. This might be the case in intensive care units (both adult and paediatric/neonatal). In such areas patients might be at high risk of infection due to their own risk factors, the presence of invasive devices and so on and so it would initially appear that, in these cases, isolation is absolutely essential. However, strict application of IPC precautions, one-to-one nursing and the use of closed circuit ventilation systems will greatly reduce any risks. As these patients need specialist care outside of their infection status, risks and benefits need to be balanced. In these cases, advice should be sought from the information provided via the IPC team.

Protective isolation

This type of isolation is carried out for the protection of the patient being isolated. Such patients are at high risk of infection and exposure to infection may be fatal when in other patients the effects would be much less severe. These are generally patients whose immune system is impaired in some way. The most common reason for protective isolation is bone marrow transplantation (BMT). It is the case that many nurses will never care for a patient in strict protective isolation as it is undertaken in specialist units and not all hospitals care for patients after BMT. It is therefore likely that you may never learn how to do this during your pre-registration, undergraduate programme of study. It may also, however, be undertaken after intensive chemotherapy (such as in acute myeloid leukaemia or in children), after some other organ transplants and where there has been severe and prolonged neutropenia and you may therefore see protective isolation being undertaken outside of the BMT setting. Sometimes it will be stated that a person needs to be placed in protective isolation but in a normal single room. In this case, air from outside the room will flow into it when the door is opened, but it is generally the case that these are patients at lower risk of infection. Putting patients in a single room is considered to improve compliance with standard precautions and it is this which is being promoted in such cases. In newer hospitals you may find rooms in areas such as the intensive care unit which can be used for both source and strict protective isolation as they can move from negative to positive pressure, depending on the needs of the patient. Positive pressure rooms are the ones used for protective isolation but once a patient is moved out of the room it will need to be changed back to negative pressure. There are strict policies and procedures in place in areas with this type of room and their use is usually monitored by the IPCT.

The psychological effects of isolation

You may think that being in a room of your own in hospital rather than in a bay with several other patients might be preferable, but not all patients feel this way. In previous studies patients in isolation have reported various feelings including loneliness, boredom, stigmatisation and even depression (Abad et al., 2010). Ensuring that we communicate well with patients in isolation is important as we quite often only go into the isolation room to carry out a physical task. Between these tasks the patient is alone and generally cannot see outside their room to find out what is going on. Psychological support is vital and we should not feel that we are not actually doing anything when we are providing such support to patients. It is also important that once a patient does not need to be isolated any longer they are either moved out of isolation or, if no bed is available, are advised that they can leave their room. This should be based on risk assessment in collaboration with the IPCT.

The next activity asks you to reflect on any previous experience that you have had with patients in isolation.

Activity 9.2   *Reflection*

If you have already been out in placement, try to remember if you have cared for patients either isolated in a single room or cohorted. What infection did the patient or patients have and how easy did you find it to look after them in this situation? Was there anything that you would do differently if you were in the same situation again? Do you feel that the patient's psychological needs were met? If you have not yet been out in practice, it is worth considering these issues when you first nurse a patient who is being nursed in isolation.

There is no answer for this activity as it involves reflecting on your own experience.

You may have thought about aspects that you did not consider at the time which is one of the values of reflecting on practice.

General points about isolation

When patients are isolated, whichever type of isolation it is, consideration should be given to the following points, so these are things to look for in practice:

- Isolation signage on the door which may include the transmission based precautions required. This will differ between organisations, so it is worth familiarising yourself with the different approaches.
- Having a clinical hand basin in the room.
- Having alcohol hand rub available outside the room.
- Having PPE available outside the room.
- Keeping the door closed (following risk assessment based on patient safety).
- Laundry and waste management.
- Management of the environment – keeping the room as tidy as possible and free from clutter – providing a rationale to patients and relatives/carers for this.
- The use of single use or single patient use equipment.
- Communication with other staff such as cleaning staff.
- The psychological effects of isolation.

Waste management

Within the healthcare setting, waste is generally categorised as either household or clinical waste. In areas such as clinics, hospitals and GP surgeries, household waste is disposed of in black bags and at patients' homes in their domestic waste bin. This covers items such as flowers, food waste and so on, though some areas now have a waste stream specifically for superfluous food. Other waste can be defined as clinical in nature and there is a need to dispose of such waste safely and correctly to reduce risk and comply with legislation. This section provides information on the colour coding system as it currently stands in the UK. However, in some organisations you will find that some of the colours are not used, as two waste streams may have been combined. This might mean that some waste is dealt with at a higher level than needed, which is not against the law, but may cost the organisation more. This is often done to simplify waste management for staff and to ensure that mistakes which may lead to prosecution are minimised.

Waste segregation and management is based on health and safety and risk assessment requirements as opposed to the principle of standard precautions and therefore, despite some organisations treating waste by standard principles, this is not meant to be the case. Disposal of waste is based on whether it is considered to be infectious or offensive. If we remember standard precautions, all patients and their body fluids are considered to be a source of infection, whether known to have an infection or not, but in waste management disposal should be based on a risk assessment. There are various terms used to define and describe waste arising from healthcare and it is therefore worth discussing some of these here so that you have a greater understanding of different categories of waste and how they should be disposed of.

Clinical waste

The Controlled Waste Regulations define clinical waste as waste from a healthcare activity that contains viable micro-organisms or their toxins which are known or believed to cause disease; contains or is contaminated with a medicine containing a biologically active pharmaceutical agent; or is a sharp or body fluid or other biological material that contains or is contaminated with a dangerous substance.

Hazardous waste

Most clinical waste is defined as hazardous. In Scotland the term 'special' is used instead of hazardous. If waste or its components can cause harm to either the environment or to human health, it is considered to be hazardous. These hazards may relate to a waste being infectious, containing hazardous medicines such as **cytotoxic** drugs, being a used sharp, or being waste arising from the care of a patient with an infection (such as an incontinence pad from a patient with *Clostridium difficile*).

Infectious waste

Healthcare staff are required to make an assessment of whether waste is infectious. This would include waste containing blood, pus or wound exudate unless nursing assessment indicates that no infection is present. This is where the difficulty arises as we are conditioned to the standard approach of assuming infection risk. If a dressing is removed from a wound and it contains blood and exudate that is not assessed to be infectious, it is not considered to be infectious waste. Neither are items used in blood transfusions.

Offensive waste

This is also sometimes referred to as hygienic waste and is considered to be non-infectious, but is waste that may cause offence due to odour, body fluids or recognisable healthcare related items. Offensive waste is not clinical waste, but can contain body fluids or excretions. It is not subject to special requirements to prevent infection. This might include items such as incontinence pads or stoma bags where the patient is not known or suspected to have a gastro-intestinal infection. It has been and continues to be the case, in particular in the hospital setting, that offensive wastes are treated as clinical and infectious waste and therefore disposed of as such when this is not necessary.

The main containers for waste disposal are bags, sharps bins and lidded sealed units. Bags are usually placed inside rigid bins with foot operated lids so that they can be opened without contaminating the hands. These come in a variety of colours which are meant for the disposal of specific items. Different colours mean that the waste will be treated differently by the waste management company after they have collected the waste from a hospital, clinic or surgery. Table 9.1 shows the containers used, how they are treated by the waste management company and gives examples of types of waste to be disposed of in these containers.

You may find in some areas that orange bags and tiger bags are not used and that all waste meant for these is disposed of in yellow bags and sent for incineration. This costs more but, as previously mentioned, is sometimes the practice to minimise the risk of an error which means that waste to be incinerated is actually disinfected instead. You may also find in some areas that orange lidded sharps bins are not used and such sharps are disposed of in the yellow lidded bin. Again, this costs more but does not contravene any legislation. This can be confusing if your placement areas differ, so each time you begin a new placement experience it is worth identifying the different colour bags and sharps bins that they use and what they dispose of in each.

When dealing with clinical waste, you should ensure that appropriate PPE is worn, that you do not decant waste from one container to another and that waste containers are not overfilled prior to being sealed and labelled.

Container	How managed	Waste examples
Orange bag	Can be disinfected, autoclaved or incinerated	*Infectious* or potentially infectious soft waste contaminated with blood or body fluids Dressings, swabs, gloves, aprons, masks, bandages and blood bags etc.
Yellow bag	Incineration only	Infectious or potentially infectious clinical waste *contaminated* with chemicals or medicinal waste IV giving sets, IV infusion bags, medicated dressings, wipes contaminated with disinfectants

(Continued)

Table 9.1 (Continued)

Container	How managed	Waste examples
Tiger bag (yellow with black stripe)	Can be disposed of in a landfill site	Non-infectious, *offensive* recognisable healthcare waste, generally items not contaminated with potentially infectious body fluids, chemicals of medicinal products Gloves, aprons not visibly contaminated with blood or body fluids Nappies, catheter bags, incontinence pads, stoma bags
Purple bag or yellow and purple bag	Incineration	Non-sharp items contaminated with cytotoxics or **cytostatics** such as swabs, classed as *hazardous*
Red lidded sealed unit	Incineration only	Anatomical waste such as body parts removed in the operating theatre, placentas following delivery
Blue lidded sealed unit	Returned to pharmacy	Out of date or patient returned pharmaceutical waste (except cytotoxics or cytostatics), empty medicine bottles, considered to be non-hazardous
Yellow lidded sharps bin	Incineration	Needles and syringes, including those contaminated with medicines (except cytotoxics and cytostatics), used medicine vials and other sharp items
Orange lidded sharps bin	Incineration, autoclaving or disinfection	Sharps which may be contaminated with body fluids but not medicinal products, cytotoxics or cytostatics such as phlebotomy needles
Purple lidded sharps bin	Incineration	For cytotoxic and cytostatic sharps

Table 9.1: Waste segregation

(RCN, 2014b)

Activity 9.3   *Decision-making*

Considering what you have learned about sharps and waste disposal in this and the previous chapter, identify what type of container the following should be disposed of in (orange bag, yellow bag, tiger bag, red lidded unit, yellow lidded unit, purple lidded unit or blue lidded unit).

a) Gloves contaminated with blood
b) A finger amputated in the operating theatre
c) A needle and syringe used to administer a depot injection in a mental health setting

d) An expired box of paracetamol

e) A needle and syringe used to administer chemotherapy

f) An empty intravenous infusion bag used to administer normal saline

g) A nappy removed from a baby on the neonatal unit

Answers can be found at the end of the chapter.

The above activity should have helped you to further clarify waste segregation requirements, in particular in hospital and clinic based settings. However, what about community nursing and waste which arises from healthcare in a patient's own home? This has presented challenges over the years and practices have varied from one locality to another. Despite nursing procedures being undertaken in a patient's home, this is classed as a place of work for the nurse and, this being the case, laws governing waste apply to both the nurse and their employer. Nurses working in the community have a responsibility to safely dispose of the waste that they produce. What this means in essence is that waste must be risk assessed to determine whether it is considered infectious or offensive, as previously mentioned.

Nurses in the community may need to arrange a waste collection service for their patients from their homes. In situations where the waste is considered to be soft and non-infectious and where the quantity is small, the RCN (2014b) highlights that this can be disposed of in the patient's domestic waste bin. The arrangements for this will vary between organisations so it is worth checking if on placement with a community nurse (in any field) how waste is dealt with. In some areas, nurses transport waste from patients' homes back to their base (such as a clinic) for disposal. If this is the case, the waste needs to be transported in UN approved packaging that is leak-proof and staff should carry a spillage kit in their vehicles. This clearly can have problems such as waste contaminating clean items in the car boot. Therefore collection from the patient's home through a collection service is the best option. This has costs for the organisation who may decide instead to put their own systems into place.

Uniform policies

Some nurses will wear uniforms in practice and some will not, depending on the area where they practice and the specific setting. For example, health visitors and community psychiatric nurses often do not wear uniforms, instead they wear their own clothes. In the hospital setting, it is more common for uniforms to be worn. Whatever is worn as a nurse, however, general principles of presentation and laundering apply and uniform policies cover issues such as health and safety and professionalism.

The Department of Health updated its initial guidance on uniforms and workwear in 2010. Its guidance has objectives related to patient safety, public confidence and staff comfort. It must be stressed here that, while we are considering infection prevention and control in this chapter, there is no conclusive evidence that uniforms play a direct role in the spread of infection.

However, the DH considers that what staff wear should minimise risks to patients, not impede correct hand hygiene and not come into contact unintentionally with patients during direct care. The basic principles of what staff wear at work are therefore identified with these issues in mind.

There is specific legislation that deals with uniforms and workwear including sections 2 and 3 of the Health and Safety at Work Act 1974, The Management of Health and Safety at Work Regulations 1999 and The Health and Social Care Act 2008 (DH, 2015). Legislation focuses primarily on health and safety including infection prevention and staff equality (RCN, 2013b).

In terms of good practice, we can consider here what should be worn, how it should be laundered and what constitutes bad practice in relation to uniform and workwear.

Whatever is worn at work, whether uniform or general clothing, such as in some mental health and community settings, sleeves should be short when undertaking clinical procedures. A clean uniform should be worn each shift and it should be changed immediately if it becomes visibly soiled or contaminated.

Uniforms and work clothing should be washed at the highest temperature allowed for the type of fabric and any heavily soiled uniforms should be washed separately from other items and uniforms.

It is considered to be bad practice to undertake non-work activities, such as going shopping, while in uniform as while there is no evidence that this is an infection risk, the public perceives one and it can appear unprofessional. Ideally uniforms should be changed into and out of at work. Where this is not possible, the uniform should be covered with a full length coat when travelling to and from work and those in uniform should not be seen in social and shopping outlets. It is worth looking at policies within your university and local Trusts to identify what is said about wearing uniforms outside work.

Activity 9.4   *Evidence-based practice and research*

If you are in university at the moment, find out whether the university (or the clinical skills laboratory) has a uniform policy. What does it say about uniform both in the skills laboratory and out in practice? If you are in a practice placement at the moment, have a look at the organisation's uniform policy. Do the staff working within your placement comply with this policy? If not, what are they doing incorrectly?

There is no answer for this activity as it involves your own observations.

The principles of asepsis

Aseptic technique can be defined as a method utilised to prevent the contamination of wounds and other susceptible sites by potentially pathogenic organisms. An aseptic technique must be used during any procedure which breaches the body's natural defences and can be categorised as surgical asepsis, aseptic non-touch technique (ANTT) or a clean technique. In nursing we utilise ANTT most often of these three.

An aseptic technique would be applied for activities such as surgical wound dressings, wound suturing, insertion of an intravenous device, insertion of a urinary catheter and insertion of a tracheostomy tube, surgical procedures and so on.

- *Surgical asepsis* is undertaken in areas such as the operating theatre where the environment is controlled with aspects such as air exchanges and so on.

- *Aseptic non-touch technique (ANTT)* involves the use of sterile items, where only sterile items come into contact with the susceptible site of the body (such as a wound). This includes any cleansing agent used, which also needs to be sterile. ANTT is applied for most wound dressing, urinary catheterisation and intravenous device management.

- *Clean technique* involves the usual standard precautions but uses clean instead of sterile gloves and tap water instead of sterile water, primarily in managing chronic wounds such as leg ulcers. This is most often used as a procedure in community settings. A Cochrane review (Fernandez and Griffiths, 2012) actually highlighted that there was no evidence that the use of tap water increased infection in even the management of acute wounds such as surgical sites but it is still the case that, in the hospital setting, acute wounds are cleansed using sterile water or saline and ANTT is applied. You may therefore never see the clean technique being applied in the hospital setting, but may see it in community and primary care placements.

As a nurse there are some aseptic procedures that you might observe and participate in on a regular basis so it is worth considering these in more detail, not just in relation to asepsis but generally from an infection prevention and control perspective. In particular, urethral catheter management and the management of intravenous devices (including central lines) are particularly important considering the burden on healthcare of catheter related urinary tract infections and bacteraemias.

The management of urethral catheters

Urethral catheters can be long-term, short-term and intermittent and while the management principles are the same for all three, there are distinct differences in practice. epic3 provides guidance for the care of short-term while NICE considers long-term and intermittent.

Whichever field of nursing you are studying, you will encounter patients who have a urinary catheter. Patients may have a catheter inserted for various reasons including:

- Urinary retention
- To bypass an obstruction
- To test bladder function

- For accurate measurement of urinary output

- To empty the contents of the bladder

- For bladder irrigation

- Incontinence following proper assessment

(Endacott et al., 2009)

Activity 9.5   *Evidence-based practice and research*

Try to find out some of the causes of urinary retention (a minimum of 5).

Some examples can be found at the end of this chapter.

Urinary catheterisation increases the risk of infection, termed catheter-associated urinary tract infection or CAUTI. Various documents highlight the contribution of CAUTI to HCAIs, identifying CAUTI as one of the most common HCAIs, not just in the UK but internationally (HICPAC, 2009; HPS, 2015; HPA, 2012). Its prevention is therefore important in the healthcare setting. Urinary catheters increase the risk of infection by enabling micro-organisms to gain entry to the bladder; by reducing the body's usual defence of flushing out micro-organisms during normal emptying of the bladder (**micturition**); and by facilitating **biofilm** formation. Each subsequent day that a catheter is in situ increases the risk of UTI until the risk approaches 100% after 30 days. Additional factors which increase the risk of CAUTI include previous catheterisation, the length that a patient is in hospital prior to being catheterised, the setting where the catheter is inserted, being female, increasing age, anatomical defects in the urinary tract, an enlarged prostate gland, conditions such as diabetes, kidney stones and sickle cell anaemia, pregnancy, the menopause, some medications and impaired immunity (HICPAC, 2009).

Activity 9.6   *Evidence-based practice and research*

Considering the factors above, why do you think being female increases the risk of UTI?

The answer can be found at the end of this chapter.

There are three main types of catheter, but various materials from which catheters can be made, each suitable for different purposes. The most common type used in nursing practice is a two-way Foley catheter which is used with patients who need bladder drainage, whether for the short-term or longer. Three-way Foley catheters are more commonly seen in urology as they provide continuous irrigation. Two- and three-way Foley catheters both have balloons to keep them inside the bladder after insertion. Nelaton or Scott's catheters are used to empty the bladder or to put solutions into the bladder (generally therefore for intermittent use). These have no balloon.

Catheters are often made from latex or latex coated with PTFE or hydrogel, but may also be made of silicone, plastic or PVC (Endacott et al., 2009).

Intermittent self-catheterisation

Where clinically appropriate and where it is a practical option for a patient, this is the type of catheterisation which should be used. It provides normality in terms of going to the toilet like other people do and having some level of control about the emptying of the bladder by the patient themselves passing a tube into their bladder to empty it, commonly into the toilet, followed by immediate removal of the tube (catheter). This is a clean rather than aseptic procedure. Most catheters used for this purpose are lubricated but when they are not, a single patient use lubricant can be used.

Long- and short-term catheterisation

Many of the IPC principles are the same, whether the catheter is for long- (up to 12 weeks), medium- (up to 28 days) or short- (up to seven days) term use. NICE (2012) and epic3 (Loveday et al., 2014) provide a set of recommendations for each which are based on the best evidence currently available. Urinary catheters should only be inserted after considering other options due to the risk of infection. Once a catheter is in situ, its need should be reviewed regularly and documented if still required and it should be removed as soon as it is no longer required.

In terms of IPC, whether the urethral catheter that is being inserted by the nurse is for long- or short-term use, its insertion is an aseptic procedure (ANTT). The type of catheter to be inserted should be based on assessment of the patient, including aspects such as allergies (such as to latex), reason for catheterisation and previous catheterisation history. The smallest gauge catheter that will allow the outflow of urine in the specific patient should be used with a 10 mL balloon in adults and a 3–5 mL balloon in children. In urology, some patients may require larger catheter and balloon sizes. There is a difference in recommendations for cleaning of the urethral meatus prior to catheter insertion, depending on whether it is for long- or short-term use. NICE (2012) recommends cleaning in accordance with local policies for long-term catheterisation which means that there may be differences between organisations. epic3 (Loveday et al., 2014) specify the use of sterile normal saline for cleansing prior to short-term catheter insertion. Both sets of guidelines recommend the use of a single use lubricant during insertion for the minimisation of trauma, discomfort and infection risk. After catheter insertion, the catheter should be connected to a sterile closed drainage system (or catheter valve) and the connection between the catheter and the drainage system should not be broken other than for sound clinical reasons. This means that at night a link system should be used, i.e. a night bag connected to the day bag, as opposed to the day bag being removed and replaced with an overnight bag. This keeps manipulations to a minimum and reduces the risk of infection. The drainage bag should be positioned below the level of the bladder and should not make contact with the floor. When manipulating the catheter, such as emptying the bag, clean gloves should be worn and clean containers should be used for each patient to empty the urine into. Catheters and catheter bags should be changed according to manufacturer instructions or if clinically indicated. When obtaining a urine sample for analysis, the sampling port should be used for this.

Suprapubic catheters

A suprapubic catheter is a type of indwelling catheter, i.e. it is not intermittent. Rather than being inserted through the urethra like the other types of catheter discussed, it is inserted through a hole in the abdomen directly into the bladder. You may see this procedure being carried out in the operating theatre under a general anaesthetic or in a more ward-based setting under a local anaesthetic. In some cases, an epidural anaesthetic may be used. This type of catheter is generally used when there is damage to or blockage of the urethra which means that a urethral catheter cannot be inserted. After insertion, the same principles apply in terms of a sterile closed system and other infection prevention and control precautions.

Documentation

It is important to document aspects relating to the insertion, care and removal of urinary catheters. How this is done will vary between organisations. As a minimum, following urinary catheterisation as a nurse you should document the following:

- The reason for the catheterisation or catheter change, or the health status of the patient prior to catheterisation.
- Initially it may be necessary to record fluid intake balanced against urinary output and in some cases this may be ongoing.
- Allergy status (for example latex, gels and medication).
- Consent obtained for the procedure; some organisations now require this to be in written form.
- If antibiotic cover was used, state drug and dosage.
- Meatal or genital abnormalities observed, including discharge.
- Whether the insertion was easy or difficult.
- Whether urine is drained, the amount, colour, smell and, if necessary, dipstick and record the result and if no urine drains, document what actions you took.
- Brand, catheter name, material, tip type, catheter length, **charrière** size, balloon size, batch number, expiry date.
- Cleaning fluid and lubricant/anaesthetic gel used.

(RCN, 2012b)

Documentation should be ongoing and might include fluid balance records and any signs and symptoms of infection relating to the urinary catheter (see Chapter 2).

Catheter care bundles/care pathways

Both nationally and internationally we have seen the introduction of care bundles and pathways in various areas of care, including urinary catheterisation. A bundle is a structured way of improving the processes of care and patient outcomes: a small, straightforward set of evidence-based practices that, when performed collectively and reliably, have been proven to improve patient outcomes. Bundles have been particularly used in central line management but increasingly bundles and care pathways have been introduced to improve patient outcomes relating to urinary catheters. The Centre for Policy on Ageing (2014) undertook a rapid review of the effectiveness of care pathways in health and social care and began by acknowledging Neuberger et al.'s (2013) point in reference to the Liverpool Care Pathway that care pathways may be an attempt to 'level up' so that individual patients and clients all receive the best standard of care available, but the counter-argument is that they are contrary to the concept of person-centred care, do not allow sufficiently for non-standard situations such as the presence of complex co-morbidities, and can become a tick-box exercise with 'too much pathway and too little care'. Despite this, the report found that there were several advantages to the use of pathways, including that they are associated with reduced in-hospital errors/complications and improved documentation without impacting on length of stay and hospital costs, generally report a positive impact on clinical outcomes, costs, patient satisfaction and teamwork, in particular the latter in enhancing cross-setting collaboration such as between hospital and community based care; and that pathways have a significant positive impact on the organisation of care. They did, however, acknowledge that most bundles and pathways are developed locally and therefore differ in their quality, scope and application. This is indicative of the various studies undertaken which reflect differences in cost benefits and patient outcomes with some identifying vast positive impacts and others no impact at all (Allen et al., 2009; Every et al., 2000). Within your clinical placements you may be asked to use a care bundle or care pathway in a variety of situations (for example there are pathways for patients with MRSA in some organisations). You therefore need to be aware that these will differ between different settings and organisations.

Intravenous device management

As with any invasive device, the main thing to remember is that they should only be used following assessment of need and consideration of other options, due to possible side effects and complications. Once it is decided that such a device is needed, there should be an assessment of the type of device that is appropriate for both the patient and for its rationale for use.

As a nursing student, depending on your placement area and the restrictions placed on student activities in some organisations, you may have no involvement or quite wide ranging involvement in the management of intravenous devices, though you will not generally be involved in insertion of such devices. It is important that you are aware of the main management principles so that if you do become involved you are able to apply the correct IPC precautions to minimise the risk of infection to the patient. IV catheter related infections can be specific to the site of the insertion of the device, so localised in nature: a 'tunnel' infection which involves the blood vessel containing the device; a bloodstream infection (referred to as a CR-BSI – catheter-related bloodstream infection); or endocarditis, which affects one of the membranes of the heart. Some such infections lead to an increase in **morbidity**, longer hospital stays and an increase in costs to healthcare organisations.

As with the sources of infection discussed in Chapter 2, CR-infection can be exogenous (caused by micro-organisms originating external to the patient such as equipment, the environment, staff etc.) or endogenous (from the patient's own body). In order to minimise the risk of intro-ducing micro-organisms into an IV site, you need to be aware of the sources and routes of contamination into the IV system. If we consider the case of a patient with a peripheral IV device sited in an arm which is connected to an intravenous infusion bag containing a fluid such as normal saline, sources and routes of contamination can be quite significant.

- EXTRINSIC contamination is that which is introduced during the use of the device and associated equipment. This might include organisms introduced by staff during infusion bag changes and during the attachment of the IV giving set to the infusion bag; via two-way taps and filters added to the infusion lines; during insertion and manipulation of the IV catheter; and from the dressing applied to the IV site.

- INTRINSIC contamination is that which is already present prior to use of the device, such as contaminants already in the infusion bag and IV giving set.

Routes of contamination are commonly referred to as:

- INTRALUMINAL (where micro-organisms are introduced directly into the IV catheter, giving set or infusion fluid via the hands of staff, contaminated equipment and bacteria on the patient's skin); or

- EXTRALUMINAL (which is when micro-organisms access the site via the outside of the IV catheter through the insertion site, again from the patient's own skin flora, dressings, contaminated ointments etc.); or

- HAEMATOGENOUS (where micro-organisms from other sites within the patient's body are transferred to the IV catheter via the bloodstream, such as wound infections and cellulitis).

(Mermel, 2011)

The risk of infection can therefore be minimised by aspects such as the correct use and stor-age of IV equipment, hand hygiene, adequate skin preparation and the use of certain types of IV lines which reduce infection. Such issues need to be considered prior to insertion and after removal of a device, ranging from the site of insertion (as some sites are considered to have a higher risk of infection than others), through manipulation and use, replacement and eventual removal.

Intravenous devices may be inserted into an artery or a vein and may be for short- or long-term use. It is likely that the one that you will most commonly see is a peripheral IV device which is for short-term use and may be used for administration of IV medication, infusions of fluids or for temporary feeding, though for the latter there are better alternatives. Organisations such as NICE and BAPEN have produced guidelines relating to infusion therapy (see further reading at the end of the chapter) which you may find useful. Types of intravenous device that you might encounter in clinical practice include:

- PVC (peripheral venous catheter) – most commonly inserted into the lower arm or hand.

- PICC (peripherally inserted central venous catheter) – an alternative to CVCs with a lower cost.

- Non-tunnelled central venous catheter (CVC) – allow simultaneous administration of more than one item and allow haemodynamic monitoring.

- TCVC (tunnelled central venous catheter) – generally surgically inserted for patients requiring long-term IV administration.

- Peripheral arterial catheter – used in more acute settings for continuous blood pressure monitoring and blood collection.

- PAC (central arterial or pulmonary arterial catheters) – larger than CVCs and generally only used in intensive care to monitor haemodynamic and cardiac performance.

- TIP (totally implanted IV port) – better for patient activity long-term but not used routinely – surgically implanted.

Both NICE (2012) and epic3 (Loveday et al., 2014) provide recommendations for IPC in the care of IV access devices. However, whatever type of IV access device is used, the number of manipulations should be kept to a minimum, hands should be decontaminated before and after manipulation, appropriate gloves should be worn, aseptic (ANTT) technique should be applied, and all equipment in contact with the circuit should be sterile.

Activity 9.7   *Evidence-based practice and research*

Go online and look at the epic3 guidelines. What do the guidelines say about the following:

1.   What type of device to use in patients requiring long-term vascular access.
2.   What the skin should be decontaminated with prior to insertion of an IV access device.
3.   What type of dressing should be used to cover the insertion site.
4.   When PVCs should be re-sited.
5.   What to use to flush and lock catheter lumens which are used frequently.
6.   How often administration sets should be changed when used for the administration of blood.

Answers can be found at the end of the chapter.

Wound management

As has previously been identified, a wound may be managed using ANTT or a clean technique. The NMC Essential Skills Clusters state that by the end of year 3, in order to register as a nurse, whatever field of nursing you have studied you should be able to 'Safely perform wound care, applying non-touch or aseptic techniques in a variety of settings'. This therefore includes both acute and primary care settings and different aseptic techniques. ANTT as applied to a wound may be taught initially in the university setting such as in a skills laboratory and the procedure to follow can be found in a clinical skills book such as the *Marsden Manual*. When out in practice you might observe slight variations in technique as different nurses might undertake a wound dressing in varying ways. This does not necessarily mean that one nurse is correct and the others are making mistakes. This is all about applying the principles of asepsis in terms of the application of standard precautions and ensuring that only sterile items come into contact with the wound (if ANTT). This includes the gloves, cleaning agent, any swabs and the dressing. This means that during the procedure these items need to remain sterile. Reading about this in a skills book gives you the steps, but actually observing it in practice is different and more useful as the staff member can explain what they are doing and why.

The aim of asepsis in wound management is to minimise the risk of wound infection. As a nurse you may come into contact with various wounds which need to be dressed using aseptic procedures, including surgical wounds, leg ulcers, pressure ulcers, wounds caused by self-harm or a suicide attempt, burns and other injuries. These all have different risks for infection. As a nursing student, when you come across these in practice you can learn a lot from the qualified nurses in terms of associated infection risks and the best management options. In this book we are considering microbiology and infection prevention and control; wound dressings and healing are other areas that you will need to learn about in relation to tissue viability, both at the university and in clinical practice. Wounds can be classified according to their cause and the stage that they are at in the healing process – an understanding of the healing process and what is involved in both acute and chronic wounds is important in understanding wound infection. Acute wounds include surgical wounds, burns and other traumatic injuries whereas chronic wounds occur when acute wounds do not heal within the expected time – these are usually associated with underlying conditions and include pressure ulcers and leg ulcers. It is likely that you will learn about the process of healing at university in a physiology related module. Wound dressings are used to facilitate this process and may also be used to treat wound infection.

It is now time for a quick assessment of what you have learned in this chapter.

Activity 9.8   *Multiple choice questions*

1. For which of the following infections should cohort nursing not be used?

    a) *Clostridium difficile*
    b) Norovirus
    c) MRSA
    d) Chicken pox
    e) Pulmonary tuberculosis

2. Which of the following items would be disposed of in an orange lidded sharps bin?

    a) A phlebotomy needle
    b) A cytotoxic sharp
    c) A cytostatic sharp
    d) A needle used to administer a morphine injection
    e) Out of date blood pressure tablets

3. At what temperature does the DH recommend that uniforms should be washed?

    a) At the lowest possible temperature
    b) At the highest possible temperature
    c) At 30°C
    d) At 40°C
    e) At 50°C

4. In which of the following cases would the application of a clean aseptic technique be appropriate?

    a) Insertion of a urinary catheter
    b) A surgical procedure in the operating theatre
    c) Management of an intravenous device
    d) Undertaking a dressing on a surgical wound
    e) Undertaking a dressing on a leg ulcer

5. How long should a short-term catheter be inserted for?

    a) Up to 3 days
    b) Up to 7 days
    c) Up to 3 weeks
    d) Up to 4 weeks
    e) Up to 12 weeks

6. Which of the following would be classified as a chronic wound?

    a) A surgical wound
    b) A leg ulcer
    c) A burn
    d) A bite
    e) A cut

Chapter summary

This has been the final chapter of this book. Throughout you have been provided with further reading and website addresses, plus have been encouraged to undertake activities to enhance your knowledge further. Microbiology and infection prevention and control

(Continued)

continued . . .

are wide ranging topics and this chapter and the book overall have introduced you to these. Throughout your nursing career you will learn more as you meet new patients and work in different settings. You may even go on to work in infectious diseases or as an infection prevention and control nurse. Whatever area you work in in the future, infection prevention will be important, from identifying your patients at risk through to the application of standard and transmission based precautions.

Activities: Brief outline answers

Activity 9.1: Reflection/evidence-based practice (page 151)

Consider the above scenario. What things do you think could have been done differently to minimise the impact of the outbreak of infection? If you are currently in clinical placement, discuss this with one of the nurses and highlight how this would have been managed in the placement area, and what factors might have prevented good management.

You might have considered the following:

- Putting patients with diarrhoea with an unknown cause together in the same room is not recommended. In this case there were two causes which could lead to cross-infection; in an ideal world patients should not have been moved together. However, in discussion with your placement you might have identified the problems with this due to lack of isolation facilities – the nurse might have said that it was the best approach to manage risk based on what was known at the time.
- Patients should not have been transferred to other wards or discharged to the nursing home. This extended the outbreak and led to closures. Staff should have adhered to what was advised by the IPCN and kept the patients on the affected wards OR moved them into single rooms for isolation in the transferred to ward/home.
- Your placement might have identified other issues such as staff being affected, allocating set staff to care for patients being cohorted so that they do not transfer the infection to unaffected patients, restrictions to visiting, difficulties with staff who visit the ward such as physiotherapists.

Activity 9.3: Decision-making (pages 156–7)

Considering what you have learned about sharps and waste disposal in this and the previous chapter, identify what type of container the following should be disposed of in (orange bag, yellow bag, tiger bag, red lidded unit, yellow lidded unit, purple lidded unit or blue lidded unit).

a) Gloves contaminated with blood: ORANGE BAG
b) A finger amputated in the operating theatre: RED LIDDED UNIT
c) A needle and syringe used to administer a depot injection in a mental health setting: YELLOW LIDDED UNIT
d) An expired box of paracetamol: BLUE LIDDED UNIT
e) A needle and syringe used to administer chemotherapy: PURPLE LIDDED UNIT
f) An empty intravenous infusion bag used to administer normal saline: YELLOW BAG
g) A nappy removed from a baby on the neonatal unit: TIGER BAG

Activity 9.5: Evidence-based practice and research (page 160)

Some causes of urinary retention include:

- obstruction at the bladder neck
- enlarged or inflamed prostate
- obstruction of the urethra (stricture)

- contraction of the urethra during voiding
- lack of sensation to pass urine
- neurological dysfunction
- urinary tract infection
- the effects of medication
- pain overriding normal bladder sensation
- psychological causes.

Activity 9.6: Evidence-based practice and research (page 160)

Why is female sex a risk factor for UTI? This is because the urethra (the tube leading from the outside of the body to the bladder) is shorter in women and the openings to the urethra and rectum are closer together in women than in men.

Activity 9.7: Evidence-based practice and research (page 165)

Go online and look at the epic3 guidelines. What do the guidelines say about the following:

1. What type of device to use in patients requiring long-term vascular access.

   A PICC.

2. What the skin should be decontaminated with prior to insertion of an IV access device.

   A single use application of 2% chlorhexidine gluconate in 70% isopropyl alcohol.

3. What type of dressing should be used to cover the insertion site.

   A sterile, transparent, semi-permeable polyurethane dressing.

4. When PVCs should be re-sited.

   When clinically indicated (not routinely).

5. What to use to flush and lock catheter lumens which are used frequently.

   Sterile normal saline.

6. How often administration sets should be changed when used for the administration of blood.

   Every 12 hours or when infusion is complete (whichever is sooner).

Activity 9.8: MCQs (pages 166–7)

1. For which of the following infections should cohort nursing not be used?

   e) Pulmonary tuberculosis

2. Which of the following items would be disposed of in an orange lidded sharps bin?

   a) A phlebotomy needle

3. At what temperature does the DH recommend that uniforms should be washed?

   b) At the highest possible temperature

4. In which of the following cases would the application of a clean aseptic technique be appropriate?

   e) Undertaking a dressing on a leg ulcer

5. How long should a short-term catheter be inserted for?

   b) Up to 7 days

6. Which of the following would be classified as a chronic wound?

   b) A leg ulcer

Further reading

Department of Health (2010) *Uniforms and workwear: guidance on uniform and workwear policies for NHS employers.* London: DH.

This is the DH document which provides additional information about uniforms in the NHS.

NICE (2013) *Intravenous fluid therapy in adults in hospital.* London: NICE.

This is NICE's clinical guideline and includes some infection prevention related standards.

Powell-Tuck, J, Gosling, P, Lobo, DN, Allison, SP, Carlson, G, Gore, M, Lewington, AJ, Pearse, RM, Mythen, MG (BAPEN) (2011) *British consensus guidelines on intravenous fluid therapy for adult surgical patients.* London: BAPEN.

RCN (2010) *Standards for infusion therapy.* London: RCN.

This is an easy to understand document which identifies basic principles in IV therapy.

Useful website

www.bapen.org.uk/pdfs/bapen_pubs/giftasup.pdf

This is a link to the BAPEN document on IV fluid therapy for adult surgical patients.

Glossary

Antibiotics: a large group of chemical substances, such as penicillin, which have the capacity to either inhibit the growth of or to destroy bacteria and other micro-organisms, used chiefly in the treatment of infectious diseases.

Antimicrobials: something which destroys or inhibits the growth of micro-organisms such as bacteria or viruses.

Antiseptic: a disinfectant that can be used on or in the body.

Auriscope: a medical instrument for examining the external part of the ear.

Bacteraemia: the presence of bacteria in the blood.

Biofilm: a thin, usually resistant layer of micro-organisms that form on and coat various surfaces such as urethral catheters and intravenous devices.

Blood cultures: a blood test undertaken to detect the presence of bacteria in the blood. It involves the use of an aseptic technique.

Bronchiolitis: inflammation of the small air passages in the lungs called the bronchioles, often the result of infection.

Budding: a form of asexual reproduction in which a new organism develops from an outgrowth or bud due to cell division at one particular site. The new organism remains attached as it grows, separating from the parent organism only when it is mature, leaving behind scar tissue. Since the reproduction is asexual, the newly created organism is a clone and is genetically identical to the parent organism.

Capsid: the protein shell of a virus.

Charrière: he was a French instrument maker.

Coagulase: a bacterial enzyme which brings about the coagulation of blood or plasma and is produced by disease-causing forms of staphylococcus.

Coliforms: a large group of bacteria inhabiting the intestinal tract of humans and animals that may cause disease.

Commensal: this is something which lives on or within another organism, and derives benefit without harming or benefiting the host individual.

Cytoplasm: the cell substance between the cell membrane and the nucleus, containing the cytosol, organelles, cytoskeleton and various particles.

Cytostatic: something which inhibits or suppresses cell growth and multiplication such as some drugs.

Cytotoxic: any agent or process that kills cells. Chemotherapy and radiotherapy are forms of cytotoxic therapy.

DNA: deoxyribonucleic acid is the hereditary material in humans and almost all other organisms.

Dyspnoea: difficult or laboured breathing.

Endocarditis: inflammation of the endocardium which is the inner lining of the heart muscle.

Endoflagella: the special flagella of spirochetes that spiral tightly around the cell instead of protruding into the environment.

Endogenous: produced within or caused by factors within the organism.

Endoscope: an instrument which can be introduced into the body to give a view of its internal parts.

Epidemiology: the branch of medicine which deals with the incidence, distribution and possible control of diseases and other factors relating to health.

Eucaryotes: an organism consisting of a cell or cells in which the genetic material is DNA in the form of chromosomes contained within a distinct nucleus.

Exogenous: having an external cause or origin.

Fascia: a thin sheath of fibrous tissue enclosing a muscle or other organ.

Fibrin: an insoluble protein formed from fibrinogen during the clotting of blood. It forms a fibrous mesh that impedes the flow of blood.

Flagella: long, thread-like appendages which provide some live single cells with the ability to move.

Flora: the collective micro-organisms in a body system.

Glycogen: a substance deposited in bodily tissues as a store of carbohydrates. It is a polysaccharide which forms glucose on hydrolysis.

Haemodynamic: relating to the flow of blood within the organs and tissues of the body.

Haemoptysis: spitting up or coughing up of blood or blood-stained mucus.

Helical: spiral shaped.

Hypoperfusion: decreased perfusion of blood through an organ.

Icosahedral: a solid figure having 20 faces.

Indigenous: innate, inherent or natural.

Inflammation: redness, swelling, pain, tenderness, heat and disturbed function of an area of the body, especially as a reaction of tissues to injurious agents.

Kinase: a type of enzyme that catalyses the transfer of phosphate groups from high-energy, phosphate-donating molecules to specific substrates.

Koplik spots: (in measles) small pale spots with reddish rims that appear on the lips and mucous membranes inside the cheeks before the skin eruption takes place.

Lipids: another word for fats, including fatty acids.

Lipopolysaccharide: a complex molecule containing both lipid and polysaccharide parts.

Lipoprotein: any compound containing both lipids and proteins.

Lysed/lysis: the disintegration of a cell by rupture of the cell wall or membrane.

Micturition: urination: the dispelling of urine from the bladder.

Morbidity: the proportion of sickness or of a specific disease in a geographical locality.

Neutropenic: having unusually low levels of white blood cells known as neutrophils.

Nosocomial: originating in a hospital.

Nucleoid: the aggregated DNA of a bacterium, seen as a distinct region inside the cell.

Pathogen: any disease-producing agent, especially a virus, bacterium or other micro-organism.

Pathogenicity: the disease-producing capacity of a pathogen.

Peptidoglycan: a substance forming the cell walls of many bacteria, consisting of glycosamino-glycan chains interlinked with short peptides.

Periplasm: the region between the cytoplasmic membrane and the outer cell membrane in Gram-negative bacteria and some Archaea.

Pessary: a medical device entered into the vagina which can delivery medication or provide structured support.

Phagocyte: a cell, such as a white blood cell, that engulfs and absorbs waste material, harmful micro-organisms or other foreign bodies in the bloodstream and tissues.

Phospholipid: a lipid with one or more phosphate groups attached to it.

Polarity: the property or characteristic that produces unequal physical effects at different points in a body or system.

Polypharmacy: the simultaneous use of multiple drugs by a single patient for one or more conditions.

Polyphosphate: a type of salt.

Prevalence: the total number of cases of a disease in a given population at a specific time.

Procaryotes: a microscopic single-celled organism that has neither a distinct nucleus with a membrane nor other specialised organelles.

Progeny virus: the offspring of a virus.

Pyrexia: a high temperature.

RCA: root cause analysis, a method of problem solving used for identifying the root causes of faults or problems.

Ribosome: a minute particle composed of protein and ribonucleic acid (RNA) that serves as the site of protein synthesis.

RNA: single stranded nucleic acids composed of nucleotides. RNA plays a major role in protein synthesis as it is involved in the transcription, decoding and translation of the genetic code to produce proteins. RNA stands for ribonucleic acid.

Septicaemia: a condition caused by pus-forming micro-organisms in the blood, sometimes referred to as 'blood poisoning'.

Sign: objective evidence of disease, e.g. blood pressure measurement.

Subcutaneous: situated or applied under the skin.

Symptom: an indication of disease perceived by the patient, e.g. feeling hot.

Synthesis: the production of chemical compounds by reaction from simpler materials.

Systemic: denoting the part of the circulatory system concerned with the transport of oxygen to and carbon dioxide from the body in general, especially as distinct from the pulmonary part concerned with the transport of oxygen from and carbon dioxide to the lungs.

Tachycardia: an abnormally fast heart rate.

Transient: lasting for a short time, temporary.

Vaginal speculum: an instrument used to hold open the vagina in certain procedures such as a cervical smear or coil insertion.

Vesicle: a fluid- or air-filled cavity or sac.

Vibrios: a type of Gram-negative bacterium, possessing a curved rod shape.

Virion: the complete, infective form of a virus outside a host cell, with a core of RNA or DNA and a capsid.

Virulent: severe or harmful in its effects.

References

Abad, C., Fearday, A. and Safdar, N. (2010) Adverse effects of isolation in hospitalised patients: a systematic review. *Journal of Hospital Infection* 76(2): 97–102.

Abdissa, A., Asrat, D., Kronvall, G., Shitu, B., Achiko, D., Zeidan, M., Yamuah, L.K. and Aseffa, A. (2011) Throat carriage rate and antimicrobial susceptibility pattern of group A Streptococci (GAS) in healthy Ethiopian school children. *Ethiopian Medical Journal* 49(3): 283.

Acheson, Sir Donald (1988) *The Public Health in England Report.* London: Department of Health and Social Security.

Agha, M. (2012) Epidemiology and pathogenesis of C. difficile and MRSA in the light of current NHS control policies: a policy review. *Annals of Medicine and Surgery* 1: 39–43.

Allen, D., Gillen, E. and Rixson, L. (2009) Systematic review of the effectiveness of integrated care pathways: what works, for whom, in which circumstances? *International Journal of Evidence-Based Healthcare* 7: 61–74.

Archer, J.R.H., Wood, D.M., Tizzard, Z., Jones, A.L. and Dargan, P.I. (2007) Alcohol hand rubs: hygiene and hazard. *British Medical Journal* 335(7630): 1154–1155.

Association for Perioperative Practice (2011) *Standards and recommendations for safe perioperative practice.* Harrogate: AFPP.

Ayliffe, G.A., Babb, J.R. and Quoraishi, A.H. (1978) A test for 'hygienic' hand disinfection. *Journal of Clinical Pathology* 31(10): 923.

Breitbart, M. (2012) Marine viruses: truth or dare. *Annual Review of Marine Science* 4: 425–448.

Brown, G.D., Denning, D.W., Gow, N.A.R., Levitz, S.M., Netea, M.G. and White, T.C. (2012) Hidden killers: human fungal infections. *Science Translational Medicine* 4(165): 165.

Centre for Policy on Ageing (2014) *The effectiveness of care pathways in health and social care: rapid review.* London: CPA.

Chan, M.F. (2010) Factors affecting the compliance of operating room nursing staff toward standard and transmission-based precautions in an acute care hospital. *American Journal of Infection Control* 38(8): 666–667.

Darawad, M.W. and Al Hussami, M. (2013) Jordanian nursing students' knowledge of, attitudes towards, and compliance with infection control precautions. *Nurse Education Today* 33(6): 580–583.

Dellinger, R.P., Levy, M.M., Rhodes, A., Annane, D., Gerlach, H., Opal, S.M., Sevransky, J.E., Sprung, C.L., Douglas, I.S., Jaeschke, R., Osborn, T.M., Nunnally, M.E., Townsend, S.R., Reinhart, K., Kleinpell, R.M., Angus, D.C., Deutschman, C.S., Machado, F.R., Rubenfeld, G.D., Webb, S.A., Beale, R.J., Vincent, J.L. and Moreno, R. (2013) International Guidelines for Management of Severe Sepsis and Septic Shock: 2012. *Critical Care Medicine* 41(2): 580–637.

Department of Health (2010) *Uniforms and workwear: guidance on uniform and workwear policies for NHS employers.* London: DH.

Department of Health (2013) *Choice framework for local policy and procedures 01-04 decontamination of linen for health and social care: management and provision.* London: DH.

Department of Health (2014) *Implementation of modified admission MRSA screening guidance for NHS (2014).* London: DH.

Department of Health (2015) *The Health and Social Care Act 2008: Code of Practice on the prevention and control of infections and related guidance.* London: DH.

Diack, A.B., Head, Mark, W., McCutcheon, S., Boyle, A., Knight, R., Ironside, J.W., Manson, J.C. and Will, R.G. (2014) Variant CJD. *Prion* 8(4): 286–295.

Dougherty, L. and Lister, S. *The Royal Marsden Manual of Clinical Nursing Procedures, Professional Edition, 9th.* Royal Marsden Manual Series. Chichester: John Wiley.

Endacott, R., Jevon, P. and Cooper, S. (2009) *Clinical Nursing Skills: Core and Advanced.* Oxford: Oxford University Press.

European Centre for Disease Prevention and Control (2007) *The First European Communicable Disease Report.* ECDC.

Every, N.R., Hochman, J., Becker, R., Kopecky, S. and Cannon, C.P. (2000) Critical pathways: a review. Committee on Acute Cardiac Care, Council on Clinical Cardiology, American Heart Association. *Circulation* 101: 461–465.

Fagernes, M. and Linges, E. (2011) Factors interfering with the microflora on hands: a regression analysis of samples from 465 healthcare workers. *Journal of Advanced Nursing* 67: 297–307.

Fernandez, R. and Griffiths, R. (2012) Water for wound cleansing. *Cochrane Database of Systematic Reviews* 2012, Issue 2. Art. No.: CD003861. DOI: 10.1002/14651858.CD003861.pub3

Ford, M. (2014) *Medical Microbiology.* Oxford: Oxford University Press.

Gordin, F.M., Schultz, M.E., Huber, R., Zubairi, S., Stock, F. and Kariyil, J. (2007) A cluster of hemodialysis-related bacteremia linked to artificial fingernails. *Infection Control and Hospital Epidemiology* 28(6): 743–744.

Greenwood, D., Slack, R., Barer, M. and Irving, W. (2012) *Medical Microbiology*, 18th edition. Churchill Livingstone.

Haas, J.P., Evans, A.M., Preston, K.E. and Larson, E.L. (2005) Risk factors for surgical site infection after cardiac surgery: the role of endogenous flora. *Journal of Acute and Critical Care* 34(2): 108–114.

Harvey, R.A., Champe, P.C. and Fisher, B.D. (2007) *Lippincott's Illustrated Reviews: Microbiology*, 2nd edition. Philadelphia: Lippincott Williams and Wilkins.

Health Protection Agency (2012a) *English national point prevalence survey on healthcare-associated infections and antimicrobial use, 2011.* London: HPA.

HPA (2012b) *Infection control precautions to minimise transmission of respiratory tract infections (RTIs) in the health-care setting.* London: HPA.

Health Protection Scotland (2014) *Guidance on prevention and control of Clostridium difficile infection (CDI) in healthcare settings in Scotland.* Available at: www.hps.scot.nhs.uk/pubs/Publication_Detail.aspx

Health Protection Scotland (2015) *National Infection Prevention and Control Manual.* Available at: www.hps.scot.nhs.uk/search/default.aspx?search=infection+manualandGo=GO

HICPAC (2009) *Guideline for prevention of catheter-associated urinary tract infections.* Atlanta, GA: CDC.

Horton, R. (1988) Linking the chain. *Nursing Times* 84(26): 44–46.

Kiser, M. and Santibanez, S. (2014) *Influenza Pandemic.* Oxford: Oxford University Press.

Landers, T., Abusalem, S., Coty, M.B. and Bingham, J. (2012) Patient-centered hand hygiene: the next step in infection prevention. *American Journal of Infection Control* 40 (4 supp 1): S11–S17.

Lloyd Smith, E., Curtin, J., Gilbart, W. and Romney, M.G. (2014) Qualitative evaluation and economic estimates of an infection control champions program. *American Journal of Infection Control* 42(12): 1303–1307.

Loveday, H.P., Wilson, J.A., Pratt, R.J., Golsorkhi, M., Tingle, A., Bak, A., Browne, J., Prieto, J. and Wilcox, M. (2014) epic3: National Evidence-Based Guidelines for Preventing Healthcare-Associated Infections in NHS Hospitals in England. *Journal of Hospital Infection* 86S1: S1–S70.

Matheny, S.C. and Kingery, J.E. (2012) Hepatitis A. *American Family Physician* 86(11): 1027–1034.

Maxmen, A. (2009) David Artis: fear no worm. *Journal of Experimental Medicine* 206(2): 262–263.

Mermel, L.A. (2011) What is the predominant source of intravascular catheter infections? *Clinical Infectious Diseases* 52(2): 211–212.

Miyachi, H., Fuyura, H., Umezawa, K., Itoh, Y., Yumiko, O., Ohshima, T., Miyamoto, M. and Asai, S. (2007) Controlling methicillin-resistant Staphylococcus aureus by stepwise implementation of preventive strategies in a university hospital: impact of a link-nurse system on the basis of multidisciplinary approaches. *American Journal of Infection Control* 35(2): 115–120.

National Audit Office (2009) *Reducing healthcare associated infections in hospitals in England.* London: NAO.

National Patient Safety Agency (2007) *Safer practice notice: colour coding hospital cleaning materials and equipment.* NPSA: London.

Neuberger, J., Guthrie, C., Aaronovitch, D., et al. (2013) *More care, less pathway: a review of the Liverpool Care Pathway.* London: Williams Lea.

NICE (2012) *Prevention and control of healthcare-associated infections in primary and community care.* London: NICE.

Nursing and Midwifery Council (2010) *The Essential Skills Clusters.* London: NMC.

Nursing and Midwifery Council (2015) *The Code.* London: NMC. Available at: www.nmc.org.uk/global assets/sitedocuments/nmc-publications/revised-new-nmc-code.pdf

Openshaw, P. (2010) Bronchiolitis. *Child Care Health and Development* 36(S1): 8.

Prajapati, A., Rai, S.K., Mukhiya, R.K. and Karki, A.B. (2012) Study on carrier rate of *Streptococcus pyogenes* among the school children and antimicrobial susceptibility pattern of isolates. *Nepal Medical College Journal* 14(3): 169–171.

Public Health England (2013a) *Immunisation against infectious disease.* London: PHE.

PHE (2013b) *Nectotising fasciitis* (NF). London: PHE.

PHE (2013c) *Updated guidance on the management and treatment of Clostridium difficile infection.* London: PHE.

PHE (2013d) *Acute trust toolkit for the early detection, management and control of carbapenamase-producing Enterobacterisceae.* London: PHE.

PHE (2014) *The management of HIV infected healthcare workers who perform exposure prone procedures: updated guidance, January 2014.* London: PHE.

PHE (2015) *Group A streptococcal infections: activity during the 2014 to 2015 season.* London: PHE.

Quattrin, R., Pecile, A., Conzut, L., Majori, J. and Brusaferro, S. (2004) Infection control nurse: a national survey. *Journal of Nursing Management* 12(5): 375–380.

RCN (2009) *Needlestick injuries: the point of prevention.* London: RCN.

RCN (2012a) *The role of the link nurse in infection prevention and control (IPC): developing a link nurse framework.* London: RCN.

RCN (2012b) *Catheter care: RCN guidance for nurses.* London: RCN.

RCN (2013a) *Sharps safety.* London: RCN.

RCN (2013b) *Guidance on uniforms and workwear.* London: RCN.

RCN (2014a) *Antimicrobial resistance.* London: RCN.

RCN (2014b) *The management of waste from health, social and personal care.* London: RCN.

Ruggeri, F.M., Di Bartolo, I., Ostanello, F. and Trevisani, M. (2013) *Hepatitis E Virus: An Emerging Zoonotic and Foodborne Pathogen.* New York: Springer.

Russell, C.D., Young, I., Leung, V. and Morris, K. (2014) Healthcare workers' decision-making about transmission-based infection control precautions is improved by a guidance summary card. *Journal of Hospital Infection* 90(3): 235–239.

Seto, W.H., Yuen, S.W.S., Cheung, C.W.Y., Ching, P.T.Y., Cowling, B.J. and Pittet, D. (2013) Hand hygiene promotion and the participation of infection control link nurses: an effective innovation to overcome campaign fatigue. *American Journal of Infection Control* 41(12): 1281–1283.

Sharts-Hopko, N. (2015) Ebola. *American Journal of Nursing* 115(3): 13.

Shenk, T.E. and Stinski, M.F., eds. (2008) *Human Cytomegalovirus.* Berlin: Springer.

Storr, J., Wigglesworth, N. and Kilpatrick, C. (2013) *Integrating human factors with infection prevention and control.* London: The Health Foundation.

Suttle, C.A. (2007) Viruses: a vast reservoir of genetic diversity and driver of global processes. *Retrovirology* 6 (Supp A): 17.

Tada, A., Watanabe, M. and Senpuku, H. (2015) Factors affecting changes in compliance with infection control practices by dentists in Japan. *American Journal of Infection Control* 43(1): 95–97.

Tanner, J., Khan, D., Walsh, S., Chernova, J., Lamont, S. and Laurent, T. (2009) Brushes and picks used on nails during the surgical scrub to reduce bacteria: a randomised trial. *Journal of Hospital Infection* 71(3): 234–238.

The Health and Safety (Sharps Instruments in Health Care) Regulations 2013. London: The Stationery Office.

Venberghe, A., Laterre, P.F., Goenen, M., Reynaert, M., Wittebole, X., Simon, A. and Haxhe, J.J. (2002) Surveillance of hospital-acquired infections in an intensive care department: the benefit of the full time presence of an infection control nurse. *Journal of Hospital Infection* 52(1): 56–59.

Ward, D.J. (2007) Hand adornment and infection control. *British Journal of Nursing* 16(11): 65–656.

Ward, D.J. (2012) Attitudes towards the infection prevention and control nurse: an interview study. *Journal of Nursing Management* 20: 648–658.

Weston, D. (2013) *Fundamentals of Infection Prevention and Control: Theory and Practice,* 2nd edition. Chichester: Wiley-Blackwell.

WHO (2009a) *WHO guidelines on hand hygiene in health care: first global patient safety challenge, clean care is safer care.* Geneva: World Health Organization.

WHO (2009b) *Glove use information leaflet.* Geneva: WHO.

Index

Note: Page references in **bold** refer to the Glossary.